WITHDRAWN

THE PALM BEACH
PAIN
RELIEF
SYSTEM

A Clinically-Proven, Natural and
Integrative Approach to Healing
Chronic Pain, Arthritis & Injuries

Daniel I. Nuchovich, M.D.

**ESSENTIAL
PUBLISHING**
N. Palm Beach, FL
www.essentialpublishing.org

Essential Publishing, Inc.
378 Northlake Boulevard, Suite 109
North Palm Beach, FL 33408
www.essentialpublishing.org
(866) 770-1916

Copyright © 2013 Daniel Nuchovich, M.D.
ISBN: 978-0-9771309-8-6

Library of Congress Control Number: 2012956129

coolingtheplanet.org

PRINTED IN THE U.S.A.

This publication was printed by a Certified Green Printer in the United States of America, providing jobs for American workers. It was also printed, with the health of the environment in mind, on recycled paper and with vegetable-based inks, and Dr. Daniel Nuchovich is planting more trees than were required to print this publication through *Cooling the Planet.*

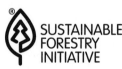

for Ana

AUTHOR'S NOTE

The author does not advocate the use of any particular form of health care but believes the information presented in this book and in his associated website should be available to the public. However, the medical information is not intended as a substitute for consulting a physician.

You should consult a physician if you think you may have a disease or a medical problem, and you should not attempt to self-diagnose nor embark on self-treatment of any kind without qualified medical supervision. Nothing in this publication or in the website is a promise or a guarantee that pain, arthritis, an injury or any other condition will disappear or improve. Nothing guarantees the safety or efficacy of any specific treatment.

This publication and the associated website are presented as educational tools to assist in the understanding, assessment and selection of treatments for health problems. I encourage the reader to consult his or her physician before undertaking any treatment. Pregnant women and debilitated individuals should not undertake any treatment mentioned in this book without the approval of their own physician.

ACKNOWLEDGMENTS

I would like to acknowledge the following people whose teaching, guidance and support were critical for this work. Without their contributions and influence this book would not be. David Eisenberg, M.D., director of the Ocher Institute of Division of Complementary and Alternative Medicine at Harvard Medical School for his vision, inspiration and leadership; Joseph F. Audette, M.D., Medical Director of the Alternative Therapy Integrative Center at Harvard Medical School, for his kindness and generosity in giving me an "inside look" at the conventional and alternative care rehabilitation center; Brian M. Berman, M.D., Director of The Center for Integrative Medicine at the University of Maryland School of Medicine for his insights and guidance in setting up an integrative care facility; Aviad Haramati, Ph.D. Professor of Education at Georgetown School of Medicine who guided me in which books to read about alternative health care. I would also like to thank Laszlo Dosa, medical writer and journalist, who assisted me in organizing and completing the first manuscript. I am infinitely grateful for my family, whose patience and kind support carried me through many long hours during the writing of this manuscript. I am extremely thankful for the love and closeness we share. In particular, I would like to thank my wife Ana. Without her, and her loving and enduring commitment to our family, this book would not be. I am humbled by her tireless dedication to this project and to the success of the *Jupiter Institute of the Healing Arts*. In spite of my cantankerous moods during the construction of this book, she remained an objective, pragmatic and focused contributor.

TABLE OF CONTENTS

Foreword xvii

✹ **INTRODUCTION:**

*Pain opened my eyes (or, how I came to found the
Jupiter Institute of the Healing Arts)* 1

   A doorway to helping others 4

   A pain program designed for you. 7

✹ **CHAPTER ONE:**

An Overview of our Pain Healing Program 9

   The seven treatment modalities 11

      1. Medical care. 11

      2. Physical therapy 13

      3. Exercise 13

      4. Chiropractic care. 14

      5. Acupuncture 14

      6. Nutrition guidance 15

      7. Supplements: vitamins, antioxidants and minerals 15

✹ **CHAPTER TWO:**

Understanding and Treating Arthritic Conditions 18

   Conventional treatment and its limitations 19

   What is arthritis? 21

      Classification 22

   Arthritis: A historic disease. 25

   Risk factors and likely causes of arthritis. 26

   Risk factors you cannot change 26

   Risk factors and likely causes that you can do

      something about 28

   The mechanics 33

      How joints work. 33

      Cartilage 34

      Joint injury, the root of the problem 36

Joint and cartilage in trouble. 37

Repair. 38

✸ CHAPTER THREE:

Understanding Inflammation. 41

A complex process. 43

The beginning. 44

The role of omega fatty acids in inflammation 45

The eicosanoid balance. 45

Fats, oils and the production of eicosanoids 47

What eicosanoids do and where. 48

Free radicals and antioxidants 50

✸ CHAPTER FOUR:

A Battle Plan for Neck and Back Pain 54

Neck pain caused by trauma 57

Neck pain not due to trauma. 59

Low back pain. 62

Sciatica and arm pain 65

The battle plan 66

✸ CHAPTER FIVE:

Understanding Common Painful Injuries 68

Overview. 70

Rotator cuff injury 71

Sprained ligaments 72

Sprained joints 73

Torn and pulled muscles 73

Bursitis 73

Tendonitis. 74

Indirect causes 75

Treating the real cause 77

Choices in treatment 78

✸ CHAPTER SIX:

Conventional Approaches to Pain Treatment 79

Conventional medical treatment 81

  Physical therapy 82

  Medications 84

    Acetaminophen 85

    Non-steroidal anti-inflammatory drugs (NSAIDs) 86

    Corticosteroids 91

    Narcotic pain killers 91

    Topical pain relievers 92

    Muscle relaxants 92

  Exercise 93

  Surgery 93

  Our Institute's approach 94

✸ CHAPTER SEVEN:

A Nutrition Plan for Prevention and Treatment 95

The avoidance plan 97

  Foods that cause arthritis, inflammation and pain 98

  Acid-forming foods 99

The Jupiter Institute Omega Diet 99

The Mediterranean Diet 100

  Key benefits 102

  The cardiovascular advantage 104

  Effects on inflammation and pain 107

More about key elements of the Mediterranean Diet 108

  Natural Antioxidants 110

  Fish and Fish Oils 111

The Jupiter Institute Omega Diet in brief 112

  Foods that are best to eat 112

  Additional recommendations for the Jupiter Institute

  Omega Diet 118

The omega-3/antioxidant state 121

The importance of what you don't eat 123

Processed foods 124

Fats: the bad and the good. 126

    The three bad fats 127

    The good fat. 128

Avoid omega-6. 128

Cholesterol and CRP 129

    To lower levels of cholesterol and LDL, the bad cholesterol. . . 129

    To raise levels HDL, the good cholesterol 129

    To lower levels of CRP 130

The anti-nutrient lifestyle 131

Pro-inflammatory foods 133

An anti-inflammatory diet. 134

Inflammation: The "Mother of all diseases"? 135

Review: anti-inflammatory foods. 137

Taking practical steps to change your diet. 138

    Pay attention to ratio of omega-3 to omega-6 140

❋ CHAPTER EIGHT:

Why Alternative Therapies Are Effective. 143

Alternative therapies that can help arthritis and

    other painful conditions 146

Official recognition 148

The Jupiter Institute Pain Program 148

Recommendations. 149

Acupuncture 150

    History. 150

    How it works 151

    Technique 153

    Acupuncture for pain, arthritis and injuries. 154

    Other indications for acupuncture. 155

    How to find an acupuncturist. 157

Chiropractic care 159

    Indications. 160

    Technique 161

    Counseling. 162

✺ CHAPTER NINE:

The Role of Supplements in Healing 163

Vitamins 167

    Cautions. 167

    Excessive vitamins 168

Cartilage-building supplements 169

    Glucosamine 169

    Chondroitin 170

    Glucosamine and chondroitin combined 171

    SAM-e 172

    MSM. 172

Minerals 173

    Boron 173

    Copper 173

    Selenium 173

    Zinc. 173

    Magnesium, iron, manganese and copper 173

    Iron. 173

    Iodine 174

Enzymes 174

    Bromelain 174

Herbs. 174

    Boswellia serratia 174

Antioxidants 174

Omega fatty acids. 175

Which supplements should I take – and how much? 177

    General recommended doses 179

    Injuries. 180

    Neuropathies and pinched nerves 180

    Arthritis. 181

    Tendonitis, bursitis and inflamed ligaments. 182

    Sizeable areas of inflammation 182

    Neck pain, back pain and chronic osteoarthritis. 183

The critical importance of choosing reliable brands. 184

Points to remember 186

■ CHAPTER TEN:

Body and Mind Exercises for Recovery 187

Act! 189

Benefits 190

Helping your muscles 192

Finding the right type of exercise for you 193

All pains are not the same! 194

Types of exercises 196

Additional information 197

Precautions and guidelines 198

Warming up 200

Tai-chi and yoga 201

Tai-chi 201

Yoga 204

■ CHAPTER ELEVEN:

"Mediterraneanizing" Your Diet 208

"Mediterraneanizing" yourself 210

Jupiter Institute Omega Diet recipes 212

Spreads 214

Pasta sauces 215

Rice 218

Salads, salsas, dressings and more 221

Meats, poultry and fish 227

■ CHAPTER TWELVE:

Weight Loss Plan 230

What you CAN eat 233

1. Protein (white is best) 233

2. Fish 233

3. Olive oil and olives 234

4. Nuts and flaxseed oil 234

5. Grains, pulses and beans 234

6. Wine 234

7A. Vegetables 234

7B. Omega-3 vegetables 235

8. Raw fruit 235

9. Herbs 235

Banned foods from the above categories 235

What NOT to eat: four enemies 236

1. Energy-dense or calorie-dense food 236

2. High-caloric meals and snacks 236

3. Processed carbohydrates and fat-free foods 237

4. Processed food (a.k.a. factory food) 238

Our toxic nutritional environment 238

More about processed carbohydrates 239

Rules 241

Narrowing your environment 243

Weight-loss Diet Menu Choices 244

Breakfast options (approx. 220 cal) 244

Midday snack (approx. 80 cal) 246

Vegetables and morning vegetables 247

Dinner (approx. 530 cal) 248

Night snack (approx. 45 cal) 252

Sauces 252

Dressings and salad dressings 253

❋ APPENDICES:

Resources for your health 262

Pain 262

Medical 263

Alternative medicine 265

Herbal medicine 266

Naturopathy 267

Schools of naturopathy 267

References 268

Index 281

FOREWORD

The Palm Beach Pain Relief System is pure inspiration! As much as it's an easy-to-understand program and expert guide for preventing and reversing inflammation and pain, this book is the compelling story of one medical doctor's triumphant recovery from a traumatic sport-related back injury and his dependency on pain-killers for managing the ensuing severe and unrelenting pain. Dr. Nuchovich's reluctant but successful graduation from the narrow-minded perspective that kept him locked in to a painful and unsuccessful course of conventional (allopathic) treatments to the expansive and healing path of natural cures serves as a wake-up call for anyone aligned with the false notion that modern medicine has the answer to pain.

What is so appealing about Dr. Nuchovich, and this book, is the frankness that he brings to the conversation about the need for wholesale changes in America's medical system, particularly in how we address pain, arthritis and other conditions of inflammation. This extremely well-educated, conventionally trained physician not only offers refreshing views about how we *need* to be living in order to avoid disease, his action of creating an *integrative medical practice* (including a chiropractor, an acupuncturist, and a physical therapist) is truly exemplary and indicative, in part, of a deep understanding of what is required for *effective* medicine.

Pain and arthritis affect untold numbers of people in America today. As I report in my book: *Reverse Arthritis and Pain Naturally: The Proven Approach to an Anti-inflammatory, Pain-free Life,* nearly 50 million people suffer with arthritis today. Another 116 million suffer from pain with an annual expenditure of $635 billion – just shy of our $711 billion yearly military expenditures!

If these statistics alone don't motivate you to read and use the extremely helpful information in this book, then consider reading this book to learn about a fine medical doctor who is practicing medicine the way it was meant to be practiced (*first, do no harm*) to celebrate the human spirit.

Dr. Nuchovich's unabashed self-characterization as a staunch, stubborn and unequivocal supporter of the medicine that he was taught (and in which he believed so vehemently), his unapologetic stance regarding numerous unsuccessful attempts at treating this pain with conventional therapies, and his genuine expression of fear and desperation when faced with the very real possibility of losing his marriage because of it, is so real and true that he inspires our compassion and self-introspection. It is this level of honesty that compels us to hear the certainty of his message, which is: *Pain and inflammation cannot be healed with conventional medicine alone; they can only be addressed successfully with a multi-faceted integrative plan where natural therapies are the focus.*

More than this, Dr. Nuchovich's authentic narration of the event – a singular visit to the office of a local chiropractor – that changed the course of his life and professional career should be enough to turn the tide of skepticism about the value of natural therapies throughout America.

Not only is it clear that Dr. Nuchovich knows and understands this subject matter inside and out, but his presentation on the process of inflammation is one of the best and easiest to comprehend that I have read. As the author of over 50 books on natural health and host of the Natural Health radio show airing coast to coast 5 days a week for the last 35 years, I know valuable material when I see it. He is thorough in his discussion of the benefits of natural therapies – in particular acupuncture, chiropractic care and physical therapy – for managing pain, and in his discussion of the necessary dietary interventions. In fact, Dr. Nuchovich demonstrates an advanced understanding – very rare in conventionally trained physicians – of the nature of our living organism when he says: "Most traditional physicians forget that joints are living tissues with cells that require proper nutrition, just like every other cell in our body." It is a discussion in which I am honored to stand with him as a colleague and comrade.

As a bi-lingual Internist holding two medical degrees – one from the School of Medicine in Montevideo at the University of Uruguay, and one from Southern Illinois University School of Medicine in Springfield, – and who also participates in ongoing training in alternative and complementary medical therapies at Harvard Medical School's Center for Integrative Medicine, Dr. Nuchovich should be commended for the tenacity with which he approaches learning, and for the passion that he brings to his patients in South Florida and abroad.

I know Dr. Nuchovich to be generous of spirit and heart, offering complimentary healthcare to migrant workers in South Florida who are largely uninsured and unable to afford care through the American system. That he has created a successful integrative pain relief program, which has improved the health and lives of 90%+ of his patients, and that he takes the time to educate and encourage his patients – regardless of means – sets this kind and caring man apart from what many of us know as "doctor."

The Palm Beach Pain Relief System is an anti-inflammatory program that works. In his gentle but direct way, Dr. Nuchovich will not only tell you *why* you must do this (if you want to be well), but give you the guidance and reassurance that you need to move forward today. This exceptionally clear and concise volume is as enjoyable to read as it is to implement, and the recipes alone make it a worthwhile manual for *anyone* seeking greater health and wellbeing for life. For those of you who are suffering from pain, arthritis and other diseases of inflammation (cancer, heart disease, and more), this book is an imperative. Not only does it provide the reasons for taking responsibility for your health and your life, it gives you valuable and proven practices that will help you liberate yourself from the shackles of pain...forever!

Bravo, Dr. Nuchovich, for this very fine contribution to the annals of health.

Gary Null, Ph.D.
New York Times Bestselling Author &
Award-winning Health Advocate

INTRODUCTION

Pain Opened My Eyes
(or, how I came to found the Jupiter
Institute of the Healing Arts)

Sometimes it takes a hard collision with reality to jolt us into an awareness of how narrowly and rigidly we view life, and our potential for experiencing it. My jolt came quite literally during a soccer game when someone collided with me on the field. I fell, and my neck snapped. It happened in an instant and at first I thought it was a minor injury and kept on playing. The next morning I woke up with some shoulder pain and stiffness in my neck. Being a physician and trained as an internist, I did what most conventional doctors tend to do when confronting pain in themselves or their patients: I prescribed pharmaceutical drugs.

As the weeks went by, the pain in the back of my neck got worse rather than better. After trying different combinations of anti-inflammatory drugs without success, I saw an orthopedic doctor. He took X-rays and suggested physical therapy. Meanwhile, I continued to take pain medication. It provided a bit of temporary relief, but at the cost of unwanted side effects. At night, I had to take sleeping pills. Even then, and after trying every bed and couch in our home, and the floor, I couldn't get a decent night's sleep or relief from the chronic discomfort.

Two months passed, and it's no exaggeration to say that during this period misery defined my entire existence. Everything I did – or did not do – was related to my pain; I became a slave to the pain. I would take a painkiller first thing in the morning so I could shower and get dressed. Then I would take muscle relaxants, anti-inflammatories and more painkillers as the day wore on. I could no longer exercise or sit to enjoy a movie with my wife. Here I was, a 44-year-old physician trained to heal others, and I couldn't find relief, much less healing, for myself. I fell deeper into despair.

Still, I continued to search for answers. Eventually, a neurologist ordered an MRI on my neck. It showed a bulging disc in my cervical spine, which was identified as the cause of my agony. The proposed solution was surgery. But that consideration scared me; I knew the sort of complications that could result from this kind of operation. I felt overwhelmed by the horror of what confronted me, and my mind kept recycling the same thought: There must be a better way, some other option, something I hadn't tried yet!

When my wife, Ana, first suggested that I turn my treatment over to a chiropractor, my reaction was immediate and indignant: "They're quacks," I snapped at her. "We were taught in medical school how unprofessional chiropractors are. What they do is baloney; it's voodoo."

Ana knew differently because she had worked as the business manager for a chiropractor. "His patients came in with pain," she told me. "But they left pain-free. I saw it happen every day."

Still, I tried to argue with her. "The guy was either cheating or giving his patients drugs or something. If they experienced relief, it might even have been from the placebo effect."

Ana remained patient, yet insistent, "No, I'm telling you. He really did help them. Besides, what do you have to lose? What are you scared of?"

I listened to her, but I just couldn't get beyond my disbelief. I was in deep denial as a result of my medical school training. I had been indoctrinated with a bias against chiropractors.

Eventually, Ana did something that shocked me. I now realize that it was the only way I could be shaken out of my intolerant and paralyzing state of mind. She gave me an ultimatum: either I would go to see the chiropractor, or she would leave me.

I don't remember ever being so scared in my life. I feared that the chiropractor's quack treatment would end up leaving me physically paralyzed, and I kept thinking that pain was better than being immobilized for life. I even had the crazy thought that I would be better off if I divorced my wife and remained married to the pain. But love and common sense prevailed, and I scheduled a visit to the chiropractor's office.

When I walked through the doors of the chiropractic clinic, I felt ashamed and hoped that no one had seen me enter. That feeling of dread was reinforced when the chiropractor came in to greet me wearing a double-breasted suit and a big smile. He shook my hand; my first impression was that I had met my executioner.

As he rubbed his fist into my ribs, I was thinking, "Oh God, I was right. He doesn't know what he's doing." I had taught anatomy classes. I knew anatomy, and it seemed that what he was doing to me would hurt me even more.

He sensed my tension; yet what he was doing was quite smart: while distracting my mind, he got me into the position where he wanted me. Suddenly, in one rapid motion, he jerked my neck. I heard the most awful noise coming from my neck and immediately froze with fear. Before I could jump off the examining table, he swiveled around and cracked my neck from another position. Then with a wave of his hand and a goodbye, he briskly walked out of the room and left me there thinking that I was going to die.

Slowly I walked out of his office to my car, with every step fearing that my neck would fall off to one side. Though I wasn't feeling any pain, I thought it was because he had broken my neck and I had lost all feeling in it. I was in shock from the surprise of what he had done to me.

As I drove my car home, the realization dawned on me that my neck wasn't broken, and I actually didn't feel any pain. My first thought was, "Shoot, this guy injected me with something." But I realized that couldn't be true. What had he done to me? What was that slick maneuver he performed? How, in four minutes, could he achieve what four months of conventional therapeutic medicine had failed to accomplish?

That night I got my first uninterrupted sleep in four months, with no pain, sleeping pills or painkillers. When I awoke pain-free the next morning, I was a believer. I didn't need to be convinced by articles or books about chiropractic medicine, nor did I need to seek approval or confirmation from the American Medical Association. I was living proof that my wife Ana was right. Chiropractors using an incredibly simple technique could be effective healers, despite what I had been taught in medical school. That four- minute experience in a chiropractor's office totally changed my mind, my career and my life.

A DOORWAY TO HELPING OTHERS

At the time of my healing experience, I was working as a specialist in preventive medicine and tropical diseases for the Palm Beach County Health Department. I soon knew, however, that I wanted to start a private practice to work with people struggling with some of the same pain issues that had afflicted me. I opened that private practice in 1993. I began referring some of my patients to chiropractors in the area on an informal basis so as to avoid problems with the Florida Board of Medicine. Most of these patients got better, as I had. My faith and confidence in exploring "alternative" ways of healing continued to grow.

My focus turned to two medical conditions that conventional medicine usually failed to treat successfully: one was painful conditions, and the other was obesity. So, I began researching these subjects and talking to other doctors who were using unconventional treatments. As a result, I decided to try acupuncture, which at that time was still being ridiculed by Western medicine as some sort of hocus-pocus technique with no proven value.

Every so often the pain in my neck would come back briefly, and I would usually go for a chiropractic adjustment. This time, I decided to visit a Chinese acupuncturist in Palm Beach County. I wanted to learn about this ancient treatment firsthand. He put nine needles in my ear and more in my scalp, and at least a dozen in my arm and my back. Then he told me to be quiet and not move. I felt an immediate relaxation come over me that deepened as the minutes passed. Half an hour later his voice woke me. My pain was gone, and my senses were alert. I had entered his office in a visual and auditory fog, and now my mind was clear. My perception of the environment was completely different.

After this experience, I continued my research into acupuncture. Within a short time, I began recommending it to some of my patients. In 2003, I attended a conference at Harvard Medical School on integrating conventional and alternative medicine. This was a pioneering conference. It showed that doorways to alternative healing were opening in mainstream medicine and that other physicians, like me, were walking through those doors. During the five-day conference, I learned more about chiropractic medicine, acupuncture, and the importance of nutrition and omega-3 essential fatty acids to health and healing. Most traditional physicians forget that joints are living tissues with cells that require proper nutrition, just like every other cell in our body.

Experts who spoke at the conference gave recommendations on when to use or combine these various approaches for the greatest benefit of patients. I learned much of value at that conference. Most importantly, I discovered that I wasn't alone, and that other conventionally trained physicians had also transcended their conditioning and opened their minds. For the first time, I began to truly understand the potential of integrating conventional and alternative medicine. I felt excited by the idea that physicians could play a role – other than pill pushers – with patients.

I was convinced when I left Boston that I was moving in the right direction for my professional career. Shortly thereafter, I founded the *Jupiter Institute of the Healing Arts*, a medical center that integrated complementary and allopathic treatments. I started by inviting an acupuncturist to come to my clinic twice a week. Next, I began searching for a chiropractor to work out of the clinic. This time, I had full confidence to do it publicly. Emboldened with approval from Harvard Medical School, I felt I could handle any challenges that the State Board of Medicine could present.

I interviewed 18 chiropractors in order to select the best one for my clinic. I went to their offices for treatment, disguising the reason for my visit as well as my credentials. I didn't feel confident with half of them and, therefore, did not request treatment. With the other half, I had them adjust my neck. Eventually, I found the chiropractor who was right for my clinic.

At first he laughed, suspicious that my offer was some sort of legal trap. I convinced him, however, that I was serious, and then proceeded to set up a room for him at the clinic. Next, I brought in a physical therapist. Finally, I had put the team together, and we began to coordinate the care of our patients. Meanwhile, I continued to study nutrition and anti-inflammatory diets, focusing on the way omega-6s and free radicals damage the tissues of the body and inhibit the healing process.

Since our clinic opened in 2003, we have successfully treated hundreds of people who had been unable to find pain-relief from conventional medicine, or had been unable to break free from the pharmaceutical drugs that were treating the symptoms but not the cause of their pain. I cannot claim that we succeed with 100 percent of our patients, but I can honestly tell you that 90 percent of them improve in significant ways when following our pain-relief program.

What we are doing is not to be considered extraordinary or far outside the norm. Experimentation is what doctors are supposed to do. They need to be willing and sufficiently open-minded to use any techniques that work – ones that enable their patients to heal and feel better. We have simply found a combination of natural, non-invasive treatment strategies that offer the greatest improvement in pain relief. The bonus is that they cost less, have the fewest side effects, and help our patients in the shortest amount of time.

A Pain Relief Program Designed For You

Now, with this book, ***The Palm Beach Pain Relief System,*** you have access to our pain-relief program without having to pack your bags and travel to our clinic in Florida.

If you are suffering from arthritis, bursitis, tendonitis, inflammation, or painful injuries of any sort, the information in these pages will help you avoid unnecessary prescription drugs and take control of your healing. I will guide you through our pain-relief program step by step. For instance, nutrition is an often overlooked component of the healing process. In this book, you will learn about the importance of diet in pain prevention and pain relief, specifically which foods and vitamins can relieve inflammation and which can stimulate inflammation and undermine health.

This book and its program are rooted in possibilities and theories, but also in the excellent results that we have seen achieved at our clinic. We don't issue disclaimers to our patients, saying "This may work." We feel confident to say that our treatments do work, and we have a track record of results as proof. In fact, there are others accomplishing similar results. My colleague Gary Null, Ph.D., internationally renowned health advocate and pioneer in the field of nutrition and optimal wellness, recently completed a program in which 50 individuals currently under the care of a physician for arthritis took part in a 4-week anti-arthritis, anti-inflammation program similar to the one outlined in this book. More than 80% of the participants realized improvement in pain and arthritis symptoms.

What also makes this book and its program unique is my own personal experience with injuries and pain. It is the foundation for much of the advice I am offering you. Not only did I suffer – and then recover from – a bulging disc, as I have described, but I have had knee and ankle injuries (both soccer-related), a hip and hamstring problem (intense gardening), and shoulder and arm trouble (from playing basketball). I have also experienced tendonitis and bursitis in my elbow and arm (improper weightlifting), and a sprained forearm and wrist (the result of an encounter with a shark!). I have had more than my share of injuries and experienced all kinds of therapies. Consequently, I can say with authority that I know what works. I also understand and empathize with the pain and suffering that you might be experiencing.

My message is that you don't have to live with the pain. Nor do you need to remain dependent on a continuous cycle of drugs and suffer from their side effects. If you have seen three or four doctors and have been prescribed a half-dozen or more medications without being cured, you are probably experiencing a range of side effects that may include insomnia, indigestion, constipation, and many more conditions that can be as debilitating as the pain condition itself. I will show you how to break that deadly cycle.

By treating the cause – rather than symptoms – of the pain in your joints, muscles, or tendons and ligaments, you can reverse the damage. You can also experience an overall improvement in health, both now and in the long run.

There is a catch, however, and you probably know what it is. You must want to do it! Instead of passively taking the pills your doctor gives you, you need to take a proactive attitude and assume responsibility for staking out your own path to wellness.

Among many other aims in writing this book, I want the healing experiences of others to inspire you to step beyond your own belief system, much as I did in abandoning the rigid mindset of conventional Western medicine. You have the inherent potential to heal yourself of the ailments that cause you pain. This book and the pain relief program outlined within it provide you with the tools to improve the quality of your life. Now is the time to begin that journey!

CHAPTER ONE

An Overview of Our Pain Healing Program

 In many ways, Amelia is typical of patients who come to us after being unable to find pain relief using conventional treatments and pharmaceutical drugs. She worked as a waitress and at the age of 45, after a decade of constantly being on her feet, had developed a progressive and debilitating pain in her right hip that threatened her mobility and her livelihood.

She had seen an orthopedic doctor, and his X-rays of her hip showed a degenerative joint disease. She took anti-inflammatory medications, cortisone shots, and two types of painkillers. The pain continued to intensify to a point where she had to cut down on the number of hours she worked at the restaurant. The loss of income undermined her ability to continue paying for the health insurance that was financing her treatment.

When Amelia arrived at our clinic, she was extremely worried about her future. The eight months of non-stop pain in her hip had triggered a series of setbacks in her life that, if unchecked, could result in her ending up dependent on welfare and the generosity of others. Not only was her health at stake, but her independence, freedom and self-esteem.

During my consultation with her, she expressed skepticism about our treatment plan because it was so unfamiliar to her. "Are you sure this will work?" she asked.

"We treat the causes of problems, instead of just covering them over with painkillers," I explained. "Too many physicians just treat symptoms. I know because I was trained that way." When I told her about my own experiences with pain and healing, it seemed to alleviate her concerns, and she confessed that she felt so desperate she was willing to try anything.

When I examined Amelia, I discovered that she had advanced degenerative disc disease between her vertebrae and sacrum (tailbone). Additionally, she had a pinched nerve in the vertebrae that put the muscles of her right hip under tension, creating friction that had led to arthritis and bursitis. As a treatment regimen, I prescribed two sessions with our chiropractor followed by a session with the acupuncturist, to be repeated after several days. In the meantime, I started her on B-complex, which is a supplement combination of B1, B2, B6 and B12 vitamins that facilitate the nourishment and healing of nerves.

Within three weeks, the severity of Amelia's pain had diminished by half. By the end of the month, her symptoms had decreased so significantly that she was able to work long hours at her waitressing job again. She continued treatment with our chiropractor and acupuncturist, seeing them just once a month, and was able to relinquish her medications. The quality of her sleep and her general health improved vastly, and she felt she had been given a new lease on life.

Amelia's case illustrates the goal of the *Jupiter Institute of the Healing Arts* program to treat pain, arthritis and injuries: to provide the fastest possible relief with the fewest possible treatments. Each patient we see is evaluated based on seven approaches that we have integrated into a comprehensive treatment plan.

Some of our treatment modalities fall within conventional medicine – for example, general medical care, nutrition and diet counseling, physical therapy, and the use of medications. We combine these with alternative medicine therapies provided in the office: acupuncture, chiropractic care, and vitamins and nutritional supplements. Alternative medicine is a term that covers all unconventional therapies and refers to medical practices or remedies outside of mainstream conventional medicine. The terms "complementary medicine" and "integrative medicine," on the other hand, are used to describe treatment programs that combine conventional medicine with alternative medicine.

The aim is to provide the best of each world, using whatever treatment is most appropriate for the individual. This is the medicine of the new century, and it is practiced by open-minded physicians who admit the limitations of their own practice and accept the knowledge of alternative medicine practitioners. This is the medicine we practice at our *Jupiter Institute of the Healing Arts* (www.jupiterinstitute.com). We combine conventional Western medicine with alternative therapies, the combination of which has proven successful in the treatment of pain, injuries and arthritis. We also encourage exercise as part of the treatment program. We follow the guidelines of Harvard Medical School, the National Institutes of Health and the major textbooks of medicine.

THE SEVEN TREATMENT MODALITIES

1. Medical Care

Medical care is provided by a doctor who maintains a dialogue with the patient and finds out about his or her problem. After a physical exam comes the evaluation of X-rays. A decision is then made about whether to perform blood tests and review old records. On occasions, an MRI or a consultation with a neurologist or an orthopedist is needed. Once the condition of the patient is properly diagnosed, a plan of treatment is discussed. As part of this conventional medicinal approach, medications such as non-steroidal anti-inflammatory drugs (NSAIDs) and painkillers may be given as a trial or for a short course. I explain the variety, use and indication of these medications in Chapter 6. NSAIDs and painkillers are good, effective and reliable only as long as they are given in short courses and as long as they are not the entire treatment, but rather a part of it. As with all pharmaceutical drugs – whether prescribed or over-the-counter (OTC) – there are risks, NSAIDs included. The primary risks in this case are kidney damage and stomach problems including ulceration and internal bleeding. In fact, about 15,000 people a year die from NSAIDs, so if you have been taking these drugs for a while, it is well advised for health sake to seek alternatives.

The medical doctor is also a member of the team of professionals that I describe here. In our clinic, the medical doctor is the team leader, but our chiropractor – and others I know – would be excellent team leaders as well. As part of his functions, the medical doctor interacts with the chiropractor, acupuncturist and physical therapist, coordinating medical management – not on paper, but in person.

Very frequently in our institute I, as the medical doctor, meet with the patient, the physical therapist and the chiropractor or acupuncturist to explain the patient's condition, review the X-rays jointly, and coordinate an integrated plan of care. These meetings are short and to the point. Some are for follow-up, to see how the patient is doing, adjust treatment, withdraw medications, assess the need for further X-rays and reports, or simply maintain the dialogue with the patient. On occasion, patients bring their relatives to meetings, and we may discuss other issues like exercise, nutrition and supplements to complement our treatment.

2. Physical Therapy

Using his knowledge and experience of the various treatment approaches, our physical therapist tailors an individual treatment plan for each patient. Physical therapy assists the healing of tender joints, sprains, tendonitis, arthritis, injuries, painful areas, inflamed muscles, and neck and back pain. The effect of physical therapy in improving function, decreasing pain and swelling, and stimulating healing is simply tremendous. (The various possible treatments are described in more detail in Chapter 8.)

I believe in physical therapy, not just because I have studied it but because I have benefited from it. As I mentioned in the introduction, I have sustained a wide variety of sports and other injuries over the course of my life. Throughout these years, I have applied physical therapy to every joint of my four limbs, so I know well how effective it is. There is no substitute for physical therapy: it is an essential part of any pain, arthritis and injury program. Our physical therapist has three attributes essential to any program like ours: he is an excellent professional, he is a team player and he is a very kind person.

3. Exercise

Much has been written about the benefits of exercise. Suffice it to say here that exercise is a fundamental part of the healing process and a healthy life. We look at exercise in more detail in Chapter 10. Although a patient without a specific complaint can pick his exercise of choice, those who suffer from arthritis and injuries cannot. They are limited to the type, frequency and intensity of exercise they can perform. Improper exercise can increase damage in the problem area. Even exercise of the right type performed too frequently or too intensively can be harmful.

A five-mile daily walk for a person with a knee problem, weight-lifting for someone with tendonitis of the arm, a tennis match for someone who already has bilateral elbow and wrist strains, or a sport activity for someone with an ankle sprain or ligament disease of the feet, are all unwise. Exercise instruction is, therefore, part of our program. It is given by the members of our team, mainly through short meetings between the patient, the chiropractor and the physiotherapist.

4. Chiropractic Care

Chiropractic treatment is very effective. It eliminates pain and restores normal function by correcting imbalances of the spine, joints and muscles. To understand what a chiropractor does, first read Chapters 2 and 4. These chapters explain how some arthritic conditions, joint disorders, injuries and nerve conditions are caused by abnormal mechanics of vertebrae and discs: alterations in positions and biomechanical structure of these vertebrae and ligaments of the spine can squeeze nerves, irritate muscles and joints, and cause damage in other parts of the body. Then read the section on chiropractic care in Chapter 8 to understand how a chiropractor works. After reading these sections, you will understand that chiropractors do for people what no other profession can.

Our chiropractor is not only extremely effective, but he is also a team player. He coordinates care with me and the physical therapist, discusses nutritional issues and exercise with me and the patient, and reviews X-rays, MRIs, reports and medical records. He talks to our acupuncturist to coordinate treatment and is an essential provider in our Jupiter Institute Pain Program.

5. Acupuncture

This wonderful healing system modulates the flow of energy in the body, enhancing its ability to heal itself. This complex but very effective treatment is described in detail in Chapter 8.

Like all of us at the Institute, our acupuncturist is a team member, coordinating patient treatments and management with me and our other therapists.

6. Nutrition Guidance

To understand our nutritional approach, you must first learn about the process of inflammation in arthritis (Chapter 2) and inflammation (Chapter 3) in general. Whether it exists in joints, tendons or spinal muscles, inflammation is complex. There are many factors, interactions and substances that create inflammation. Omega-3 and omega-6 fatty acids, free radicals, antioxidants and eicosanoids all play a role in the process of inflammation. You can affect these factors by adjusting your nutrition. Your diet can make your arthritis, injury or painful joints worse or better. The Jupiter Institute Omega Diet, which we consider a healing diet, is explained in Chapter 7. This diet provides plenty of good omega-3 fatty acids and multiple antioxidants, reduces intake of bad omega-6 and free radicals, and promotes the healing of damaged tissue.

Our patients receive nutritional guidance along with all the other therapies.

7. Supplements: Vitamins, Antioxidants and Minerals

High-quality nutritional supplements are recommended to boost the level of antioxidants and omega-3 fatty acids in the body. These and other supplements, such as glucosamine, work on the damaged areas of joints, ligaments, tendons and muscles to promote healing. Again, the chapters on arthritis and inflammation will help you understand why taking supplements will tip the healing scales in your favor. Detailed information on vitamins and supplements is provided in Chapter 9.

For those who want to learn more about acupuncture, chiropractic care, nutrition and vitamins, look for our up-to-date list of recommended reference books on our website (www.jupiterinstitute.com). You can obtain books listed on our website from your library or bookstore. However, if you are searching for a particular book and cannot find it, fax me your request to (561) 744-5349, or e-mail your question to me at (Igal50@aol.com).

We do not have a preset therapy program where every patient gets the same treatment. Every aspect of treatment is decided according to the needs of the individual patient. In some patients, nutritional adjustment and acupuncture have priority, while in others, physical therapy and medications are the first step. Some patients are candidates for chiropractic treatment, some are not. Whether NSAIDs are prescribed and for how long; whether glucosamine, omega-3 capsules, vitamins or other supplements are given; and whether dietary or nutritional adjustments are emphasized are decided according to the patient's condition. We take into account that not every therapy suits every person.

The brand of vitamins and supplements is another factor that affects success. Most brands of glucosamine, omega-3s, vitamins and supplements are unreliable; the capsules do not contain what is written on the label and may actually make the treatment unsuccessful. Some dubious brands may even contain impurities. Only a few brands of vitamins and supplements contain high-quality ingredients. Consult your physician and chiropractor, our website (www.jupiterinstitute.com) or the manager of your local health-food store for recommended brands.

Wherever we deem it necessary, we advise patients regarding other conventional and alternative treatments including injections, consultations with orthopedic doctors or neurologists, and herbal medicine.

A word of caution: I would like to emphasize that this same combination of therapy and professionals may not work in every setting. Not every acupuncturist is helpful, not all chiropractors have suitable technique, and some medical doctors and physical therapists are not the right ones for the job. Conversely, the professionals might be qualified but may not be good team players. Hence, this integration may not work in other centers.

Let me give you a few examples: Two cooks do not necessarily make a good meal; five good basketball players do not always make a great team; and a bunch of nurses and doctors do not necessarily make a good clinic. Some emergency rooms are a mess, while others are wonderful. Why? Is it because of a particular doctor or a special nurse? Or, because the doctors, nurses and support staff make a good team? Yes, teamwork is the answer. And it is more than working side-by-side. Teamwork is more like "liking-respecting-helping" each other.

This combination of conventional medicine with the best of alternative medicine is called *integrative medicine,* and it works! This approach, now encouraged by the best medical schools and the National Institutes of Health, focuses on tackling the root cause of a patient's problem rather than masking it with pills. In multidisciplinary integrative medicine centers like the *Jupiter Institute of Healing Arts,* a team of doctors, chiropractors, acupuncturists, physical therapists and nutritionists work together and offer patients a variety of treatment choices. This integration decreases or eliminates prescription drugs, avoids long waits for appointments with specialists, and gives the patient the freedom to coordinate his or her own care.

CHAPTER TWO

Understanding and Treating Arthritic Conditions

 With advancing age, most of us will experience some degree of manageable arthritic pain in some part of our body. However, there are those like my colleague Gary Null, Ph.D. who believe and promote that even this is a matter of choice, and that much of arthritis can be avoided with proper measures, such as those outlined in this book. When arthritis becomes a degenerative condition, however, treating only the symptoms rather than the causes can totally alter the quality of one's life.

Sonia, a 75-year-old widow and grandmother, came to us in a wheelchair. She had a degenerative disc disease that was affecting her ability to walk. She was taking numerous medications, including painkillers and drugs for diabetes and high blood pressure. She had seen a neurologist, an endocrinologist and an orthopedist. But no one and nothing seemed to improve her condition. The first thing I noticed from her blood tests was that she was seriously deficient in B12 and B6 vitamins. Immediately, we put her on vitamin supplements and changed her diet radically from the fatty,

meat-centered diet she typically ate to a nutrition-rich Mediterranean-type regimen. She also began chiropractic treatments once a week, followed by acupuncture sessions, and physical therapy exercises that she could do at home.

Little by little, Sonia's condition improved. After one month, she no longer needed a wheelchair, just a cane for walking support. She began sleeping better, her pain diminished significantly, and her coordination and mobility continued to improve. After two months, she was walking without the cane and had dispensed with the pharmaceutical drugs, taking only Tylenol for the occasional pain flare-ups. By the third month of treatment, her vitality had returned and she was taking overseas trips.

CONVENTIONAL TREATMENT AND ITS LIMITATIONS

Millions of people suffer from pain, arthritis, bulging discs, injury, or from all four. The standard medical treatment has simply been to prescribe medication to reduce the symptoms, such as anti-inflammatories (Advil, Aleve, Ibuprofen, Naproxen, Celebrex, Vioxx, Bextra, Indocin, etc.), muscle relaxants (Soma, Skelaxin, Parafon, Valium, etc.), and pain medications (Tylenol, Darvocet, Lorcet, Codeine, Percocet, etc.). These pills just supply a "mask of relief." Because the sources of the problem – cell damage and tissue degeneration – are not being treated, the damage worsens.

As the joint or part of the body deteriorates, more medications are needed and new prescriptions are given. Increase the white pill from twice a day to four times a day, the red tablets from two to three times a day, and so on. Very often, the doctor dismisses the patient with a pat on the back and one or two prescriptions, saying "I'll see you in a month." Soon the patient is taking three or four different medications. As he or she continues to complain, more professionals become involved in care, including perhaps a rheumatologist, an orthopedic surgeon, a neurologist, a pain clinic specialist and sometimes even a psychiatrist. Injections and steroids will follow sooner or later. Sleep or the digestive system may be affected, so an appointment with a sleep clinic or gastroenterologist may be the next step. Lab tests and X-rays will be done as well. As the condition fails to improve and as pain persists, patients become overwhelmed with medical appointments and pills. They lose their independence, become slaves to their condition, and find themselves trapped in the maze of the medical system.

Pain relief is important, of course. But the failure to treat the cause means that the painful condition will progress. In the end, surgery appears to be the only possible solution. However, even if the surgery is successful, the deterioration of the tissues may have progressed so far that pain and disability persist and the freedom the patient seeks remains beyond reach.

If you could look back and see the evolution of your suffering joint, or of the joint of your spouse, parents or relatives, you would observe something like a slow motion picture of progressive degeneration. This very slow deterioration will have been years in the forming, with the joint tissues slowly but surely affected by the process we describe in this chapter.

As you read this, ask yourself: "Why has the doctor just kept giving me pills and pain killers and done so little to actually improve the joint all those years?" And, "Why was an orthopedic doctor consulted so many times while he just kept switching pills and giving those cortisone shots, to no avail?" Or, "Why have none of these highly trained specialists ever told me to try something unconventional or pursue an alternative course to prevent the joints from wasting away like this?"

Here are two even more interesting questions: "What could have been done three or four years before that joint deteriorated so badly to stop its degenerative wasting?" I want you to remember this question, and the second: "What can be done today so that in one or two years the problem joint will cease being a problem?"

I'll tell you what can be done: First, understand the process of arthritis, injury and pain. Look for the answer in this book and perhaps in one or two additional books found in the bibliography at the end of this volume or mentioned on our website. Then accept that conventional medicine alone is not enough to take care of these problems. Be receptive to alternative medicine options. Then develop an active attitude and assume responsibility for being the caretaker of your joints.

As a starting point, we are going to explain the process of arthritis.

WHAT IS ARTHRITIS?

Arthritis, properly called osteoarthritis, is a degenerative joint disease marked by the breakdown of the cartilage in the joints. This breakdown of cartilage leads to swelling, stiffness and pain. It usually affects the surrounding tissues of the joint, involving muscle, tendons and ligaments. As the disease progresses, the cartilage thins and ulcerates (forming small tears or holes), abnormal calcifications occur, spurs grow, and the function of the joint declines. As joint movement becomes increasingly restricted, stiffness, pain and swelling worsen. Finally, the joint becomes crippled and disabled.

The term "arthritis" is used generally to mean a painful swelling in a joint, without indicating any particular cause. Indeed, the term covers a large group of conditions of different types, which include back pain, hip pain, neck pain, rheumatoid arthritis, bursitis, injured joints, ligament injuries, metabolic joint diseases and many other joint conditions.

Let's clarify this: If your elbow is hurting and you call it arthritis, then yes, it may be osteoarthritis, but it may also be tendonitis, bursitis, ligament sprain, rheumatoid arthritis or the inflammatory manifestation of a general disease. Osteoarthritis is just one of the many painful conditions that can affect the elbow.

Similarly, a painful knee may or may not be due to osteoarthritis. Numerous conditions such as ligament or tendon injuries, gout, and even infections can cause the knee joint to swell and hurt, but they are not osteoarthritis. We use the term arthritis as a general way of saying that a particular joint is sick. But if we want to establish a classification that will help with management and treatment, we need to determine the type of condition we are facing.

Classification

For proper treatment, arthritis needs to be separated into two main groups: Group A, the arthritic conditions caused by a local injury, and Group B, the arthritic condition caused by a general (whole-body) disease. Since this division determines the type of treatment, it is extremely important to understand it.

In **Group A,** local causes such as injuries, usage, posture, sprains, trauma, etc. cause localized pain, heat and swelling, which in turn causes inflammation of the ligament, tendons, muscles and joints, and degeneration in knees, neck, fingers, wrists, shoulders, hips and spine. **These conditions are the focus of this book** and they need to be separated from those in Group B.

Group B includes the joint conditions caused by the effect of a general disease, such as rheumatoid arthritis, lupus, vasculitis, psoriasis, and immune or metabolic disorders. In these disorders, the joint pain is just one of the general body manifestations of a whole-body disease.

Hence, when confronting an achy joint, unless the cause of the ache is very clear, the first step in management is to decide whether the condition is in the A or in the B group – whether the cause is local or general. This decision can be made only through evaluation and an examination by a physician who may also order X-rays and lab tests. Many people do not like to go to doctors – or they do not trust them (and even though I am a doctor I understand this) – but there is just no other way to accomplish a proper diagnosis.

Most general diseases show abnormal laboratory results that help in the identification. Many also show specific radiological findings that will aid in the diagnosis. If medical evaluation shows that a problem joint is related to a general disease (Group B), as described above, the patient needs to be seen by a medical specialist without delay. General diseases such as lupus, rheumatoid arthritis, metabolic diseases and infectious joint disease require complex medical treatment. However, the effects of these diseases can be significantly reduced – and even potentially eliminated – by implementing the many lifestyle suggestions in this book, so please read on.

In this chapter, we will be addressing the arthritis conditions due to local causes – Group A – which are by far the most frequent. Nevertheless, this initial classification in Group A or B is critical. A painful joint should always be evaluated by a qualified physician. Once this step is taken, and Group B arthritis has been ruled out, then adequate treatment can be initiated to deal with the sick joint.

Group A: Local causes of arthritis

- Bursitis
- Cartilage or meniscus injury, or inflammation
- Degenerative joint disease (osteoarthritis)
- Infectious arthritis (bacteria, fungus, virus)
- Tendonitis
- Tenosynovitis
- Trauma

Group B: Systemic diseases that cause arthritis

- Cancer
- Connective tissue diseases
- Endocrine disease (diabetes, hyperparathyroidism, thyroid disease)
- Juvenile arthritis
- Lupus erythematosus
- Lyme disease
- Metabolic disease (gout, pseudo-gout, etc.)

- Neuropathies
- Polymyositis
- Psoriasis
- Rheumatoid arthritis
- Vasculitis

As you can see, "arthritis" in a finger, ankle, elbow or hip may be the result of multiple conditions. If your neighbor complains of arthritis, the question to ask is "What kind?" Arthritic conditions should be referred to in the plural because they encompass more than 100 different diseases. Arthritis takes many forms and osteoarthritis is just one of them.

Pain in a joint, as noted previously, may be caused by an injury to any of the joint's structures: cartilage, ligament, tendons or bursa. A wrist may hurt because of irritation in the tendon passing through it (tendonitis), or a finger may hurt due to a sprain in the ligament. A shoulder may hurt due to the swelling of one of the bursa (bursitis), a sprain in the tendon, or a muscle tear. A knee may swell and hurt due to both a hurting ligament and tendonitis. You get the idea. All these conditions may trigger pain in the joint, but they are not true osteoarthritis. They are tender, swollen and hot, yes, but they are not osteoarthritis because they are *outside the joint.*

True osteoarthritis or degenerative joint disease affects the inside of the joint, involving the cartilage and bones of the joint, and the structures of the joint space. This is the most frequent type of arthritis; it is indeed a true arthritis and one of the main subjects of this chapter.

So, let us review. A painful joint (shoulder, knee, wrist, etc.) may be due to:

- an arthritic condition caused by a general disease.
- an arthritic condition caused by a ligament sprain (tendonitis, spur or bursitis).
- osteoarthritis of the joint.
- a traumatic injury to the joint caused by a sport, accident or work.
- pain and swelling caused by infection or growth.

Each of these conditions results in a painful joint (wrist, knee, etc). People may refer to them all as arthritis – a general term that is easy to remember – but each one of them is different and requires a different type of treatment. It is through medical evaluation that the appropriate type of therapy can be determined.

ARTHRITIS: A HISTORIC DISEASE

Arthritis has been affecting people for a very long time. The ancient Greeks knew about it. In fact they gave us the word to describe the condition: from *arthros,* meaning joint, and *itis,* meaning inflammation. The Romans were familiar with arthritis as well. A historian has estimated that more than 70 percent of Romans over the age of 30 were afflicted with some form of arthritis. One of the functions of the famous Roman baths was to help ease the aching joints.

Books on the subject started to be written as early as the 16th century, and by the mid-17th century many books on arthritic conditions were available. Over the centuries, countless people have suffered from arthritis. One of the most famous was the French impressionist Pierre-Auguste Renoir, the man who painted the beautiful *Luncheon of the Boating Party* in 1881 and the *Dance at Bourgival* in 1883. Renoir was born in 1841 and lived until 1919, but his best paintings all date from the 19th century because for the last 20 years of his life his hands were severely crippled with arthritis.

The last 50 years have brought major advancements in the classification, management and treatment of arthritis. Now, arthritis can be better understood and treated, providing relief and improvement in the quality of life.

Research continues in many different fields of arthritis, including immunology, genetics and microbiology, in an effort to find the mechanisms of joint inflammation and deterioration. Better understanding will lead to new and better treatment.

Risk Factors And Likely Causes Of Arthritis

Now we begin the interesting part. Understanding the causes of arthritis will help you see that many of these factors can actually be modified. Yes, you can change (and sometimes even eliminate) some of the causes of your own arthritis.

The exact cause of arthritis is not very clear. We know it happens, but we don't know why. Physicians know that physical injury such as an ankle sprain or ligament trauma can set the stage for arthritis; these injuries affect wear and tear on the joints. Repetitive trauma is also considered being among the causes.

However, many publications show that degenerative joint disease is not just a passive ulceration in the cartilage but rather an active biochemical process that adversely alters the structure and repair mechanism of the cartilage and joint tissues. This is similar to what happens when you scratch a bug bite: rather than simply wearing away skin tissue, you are triggering a complex mechanism of defense, inflammation and repair.

The arthritic process begins when enzymes damage the collagen fibers that maintain the structure of the cartilage. This damage to fibers and cartilage, and the irritation caused by the enzymes, trigger the inflammatory process.

Risk Factors You Cannot Or May Not Be Able To Change

Scientists have pinpointed several predisposing factors that increase the risk of developing arthritis:

1. **Genetic predisposition.** Some people carry a genetic predisposition to developing arthritis. This means they have a gene, or a genetic marker, that makes them susceptible to the condition. For instance, if a person's parents have osteoarthritis

there is a good chance that he or she will develop osteoarthritis too. Some families are affected by the same type of arthritis in almost every generation, which clearly shows that osteoarthritis has a high heritable component.

Researchers have found that a large number of different genes contribute to the development of osteoarthritis. Defects in the gene that causes arthritis may lead to the development of abnormal proteins in the cartilage, the growth of abnormal collagen fibers, or in abnormalities in one or two structures of the joint. The genes most commonly affect either the strength or the repair capacity of the cartilage, enhancing the damaging effect of daily wear and tear.

However, there are a growing number of scientists and other professionals, with supporting research to back them, who believe that gene expression can be altered through healthy lifestyle choices.

2. **Ethnicity.** Whether or not a person develops arthritis may also depend on their ethnic background. Certain ethnic groups have shown a higher incidence of osteoarthritis. There is some evidence that Asians, especially Chinese, have lower rates of osteoarthritis in the hip but higher in the knee. African-Americans of both sexes tend to have a higher rate of osteoarthritis than other races.

3. **Age.** It is a fact of life that the risk of developing arthritis increases with age. The older the person, the more wear and tear the joints have undergone and the higher the chance of developing arthritis. The risk of developing osteoarthritis increases even more after age 45. However, as I mentioned before, you can greatly *decrease* your chances of developing arthritis by developing healthy habits (such as proper eating, regular, adequate exercise, stress reduction, and so on) early on, and maintaining these habits throughout life.

Risk Factors And Likely Causes That You Can Do Something About

While there is little that we can do about the three risk factors above, we can do something about the remaining ones:

4. **Joint abuse.** Repetitive activities performed on a regular basis over the course of many years may make a person prone to developing arthritis in a stressed joint. Whether sports- or work-related, repetitive activities cause repetitive micro-injuries to the joint structure, causing cartilage breakdown and faulty repair. This, in time, leads to joint degeneration and osteoarthritis. The affected joints in these cases will be the ones that suffer most from the repetitive activities, such as a soccer player's knee, a tennis player's elbow, a typist's wrist and fingers, or a construction worker's hips and back.

   Osteoarthritis resulting from sports injuries is on the rise as more people are exercising and playing sports in their leisure time. Sports activities that begin in the teenage years and continue to middle age carry a greater risk of causing osteoarthritis.

5. **Weight.** If a person has excess weight, which is now more likely the case than not in America, then the bones and joints must work harder to support those extra pounds. This is especially true for the joints of the hips, knees and ankles. Over time, the extra weight hammers the joint, causing damage that the body cannot fix. The degenerative process starts and progresses. As the process advances, minor daily activities like shopping or walking to the car may trigger acute joint inflammation. An obese person may engage in an exercise program and start walking half a mile or more a day. This will not be good news for his or her joints: the hammering of hundreds of pounds may cause irreversible damage to hips, knees or ankles. Studies show that overweight women are about nine times more likely to develop osteoarthritis

than women of normal weight. Overweight men are four times more likely to develop osteoarthritis than a man of normal weight. The association between body weight and osteoarthritis becomes stronger as people become heavier.

6. **Nutritional causes.** It is now understood that cartilage is not just a lifeless layer of rubber but rather a living tissue that is continually renewed. A continuous process of breakdown and repair by the body keeps it fresh and functional. Special cells in the cartilage are continuously digesting old cartilage and creating new ones as part of the joint's normal function. To make new cartilage, these cartilage-building cells need special nutrients that come from the foods we eat. Hence, the process of breakdown and repair seems to be influenced by nutrition. Indeed, recent publications report that nutritional deficits can adversely affect cartilage's biochemical and biophysical strength. Among the nutritional causes for osteoarthritis we find:

a. **Effect of free radicals.** A free radical is a damaged oxygen molecule that destroys healthy connective tissue. Free radicals are harmful to all the tissues of our body, including the cartilage, and they are generated in response to any type of stress (chemical, physical, emotional and mental). Other causes of free radicals include exposure to environmental toxins in food, air and water. Free radicals cause a very slow degeneration of the cartilage, which initially shows no symptoms. By the time arthritis settles in and the symptoms begin, however, the damage is already significant. Free radicals also hurt the "omega-3 good eicosanoid" system, explained in the next chapter, which is our bodies' tissue-healing system. The adverse effects of free radicals are twofold: direct damage to cells and the anti-healing effect.

b. **Nutrient deficiency.** Many nutrients are involved in the synthesis of cartilage. Unhealthy nutritional habits can deprive the body of these essential nutrients and cause weakness in the cartilage structure. Some of these nutritional deficiencies are caused by low intake of vitamins C and E and deficiency of boron and niacin. Certain eating habits, such as those associated with the Standard American Diet (S.A.D.) are known to cause adverse effects in the joints. The Standard American Diet, rich in fat and processed carbohydrates but poor in omega-3 fatty acids (omega-3s), is a clear contributor to osteoarthritis. Those who eat lots of fast food and no fresh salads or fruits deprive their bodies of healthy essential fatty acids and anti-oxidants. Add free-radical damage to this and you have a sure recipe for trouble.

c. **Food allergies.** There are indications that food allergies play a significant role in the onset and progression of osteoarthritis. Foods that most commonly create arthritic conditions include dairy products, beef, yeast, wheat, eggs, oranges, peanuts, green beans, vegetables of the nightshade family (peppers, tomatoes, eggplant, potatoes), chocolate, sugar, corn and yellow wax beans.

Now, please don't toss everything out of your refrigerator. Not every arthritis patient has food allergies, and those who do may be allergic to some of these food products but not to all. We suggest you review your eating habits and your symptoms and consider withdrawing two or three of those foodstuffs. We also suggest that you consider the possibility that you may have a food allergy. Your local health food stores and naturopathic physicians will usually have information on the subject, including possible testing outlets. Searching the internet may also be enlightening (although often time-consuming and sometimes misleading).

d. **Metals and minerals.** High levels of copper, mercury and aluminum are found in many patients with osteoarthritis. It is believed that their negative effects result from their interference with the absorption and use of vitamins and antioxidants. Imbalance in minerals such as selenium, boron, manganese, zinc and calcium can cause disorders in the cartilage structure. Therefore, either deficiencies or excesses of minerals and metals will lead to cartilage weakness. What can you do about it? Eat a variety of raw vegetables and fruits and, again, visit your local health food store and natural health practitioners to gather information about taking a light mineral replacement. Here again, searching the internet may be of help, subject to the same caveats.

e. **Pro-inflammatory diet.** The nutrients in the foods we eat are the body's building blocks. They are of particular importance to the immune system, which regulates inflammation. Adequate nutrition will produce a normally functioning immune system and, therefore, an adequate response to inflammation. This is accomplished through the food components known as essential fatty acids (Omega-3s, -6s and -9s). Omega fatty acids are converted by the cells into molecules called eicosanoids (pronounced ee-**ko**-sin-oids) which play a vital role in regulating the inflammatory process.

In ideal conditions, we eat a high amount of omega-3s (which produce "good," or anti-inflammatory eicosanoids) and just a small amount of omega-6s (which produce "bad," or pro-inflammatory eicosanoids). Consuming large amounts of omega-6 fatty acids and very little omega-3s and anti-oxidants (omega-3 protectors) causes inflammation. This is anti-healing nutrition, generating few of the good eicosanoids and too much of the harmful ones. In this situation, a small joint can lead to a disproportionately large amount of inflammation. The injury may then take too long to heal, or arthritis of the joint is magnified and prolonged.

7. **The indirect effect.** Arthritis may have its root in a distant part of the body, the spine. If a person has a degenerative or

inflammatory process occurring in the spine such as disc disease or spinal arthritis, the nerves coming out of the spine will be squeezed and become irritated. If an irritated nerve goes to a muscle, the irritation will be transmitted to the muscle. Then the muscle, which passes over a joint like a bridge and helps hold it together, will not work well – it will either be too relaxed or too tense, because of abnormal nerve stimulation. If it is too tense, it will squeeze the bones together, increasing rubbing and friction, causing cartilage damage. However, if the muscle is too relaxed, it will not hold the joint together, which creates misalignment and upsets the balance of the joint. The imbalance will cause an abnormal motion of the joint, which sooner or later ends up harming its cartilage and ligaments. Therefore, excessive relaxation or excessive contraction of the irritated muscle may trigger the inflammatory and degenerative process leading to arthritis. That is how neck arthritis can cause osteoarthritis of the shoulder, or spinal arthritis in the lower back can cause arthritis of the hip and knee.

8. **Combinations of factors.** Putting aside the factors (genetic, ethnicity and age) that can be difficult to affect, imagine someone with a combination of risk factors. An obese person who abuses his joints at work (thereby exposing himself to greater free-radical damage), and whose nutrition is mostly fast food (and hence generates bad eicosanoids), stands a good chance of developing arthritis. So, does a person with a bulging disc whose weight is normal but whose nutrition is deficient in vitamins and antioxidants and full of food allergens. Similarly, osteoarthritis may result from other combinations of the factors described above. In some individuals, genetic predisposition and food allergies may be more significant. In others, age and obesity will be the cause. Yet in others, a combination of repetitive sports activities and poor nutrition may be the determining factors.

THE MECHANICS
How joints work

A joint is a place where two bones come together. The connecting ends of the bones are covered by *cartilage*. This smooth, tough, rubbery material surrounds the whole head of the bone and works like a shock absorber, preventing the bones from rubbing against each other.

Surrounding the joint is a strong cylindrical sheet that attaches to the end of each bone, the *capsule*. You can visualize it by putting your two fists together inside the sleeve of a shirt. The capsule keeps the joint in a closed sterile environment and is reinforced in several areas by a thick bundle of fibers called *ligaments*. The ligaments are anchored to the bone on either side of the joint, and they hold the joint together and keep it well aligned. Ligaments are tough structures made of collagen fibers and they cross from one bone end to the next like bridges. Weakness or loosening of ligaments results in the misalignment of the joint, which accelerates joint injury.

The inside of the joint is lubricated by a thick, clear liquid called *synovial fluid,* which helps the joint surfaces slide more easily. The fluid is like oil that protects the cartilage and decreases friction. Essentially, the joint is a closed compartment where the wrapping capsule, lubricated by the synovial fluid, holds the bones together.

Tendons are fibrous cords that go from muscle to bone. They are intermediate structures that attach muscle to bone and pass through the outer part of the joint like bridges, helping to hold it together.

Outside, in addition to ligaments and tendons, and attached to the joint, we find bursas. *Bursas* are small sacs also filled with synovial fluid that sit like tiny cushions between the joint and tendons and facilitate their sliding. They are designed to relieve friction between these structures.

Cartilage

The cartilage of a joint (*articular* cartilage) is a dense, rubbery material that covers the two heads of the bones. It is whitish in color and extremely tough. Its major constituents are water, protein and fibers called collagens, all mixed together with cells to create a tissue with a strong structure. The firmness and health of the cartilage is crucial for the proper function of the spine and joints. In the painful disorders that we review here, no treatment program is complete without the management of the process that alters the metabolic harmony of this cartilage.

As we've just noted, cartilage is made of cells, protein and fibers, all packed together. The cells of the cartilage, called *chondrocytes,* are loaded with enzymes and are responsible for synthesizing the proteins. Chondrocytes are metabolically very active, and they are capable of regeneration and repair when confronted with injury. But they are also subject to auto-damage. When an injury is significant enough to burst chondrocytes open, the enzymes are scattered, resulting in damage to the surrounding tissues.

The major function of the articular cartilage is to coat the bones and absorb shock. The proteins in the cartilage act like sponges, holding water during rest and pushing the water out when under pressure. This water-in/water-out system absorbs the mechanical forces and provides important protection against the pressure of a mechanical force. This allows the cartilage to give and to flatten against pressure instead of cracking and breaking.

An important function inside the joint is the lubrication. The cartilage surface, wet with synovial fluid, is slippery, allowing the joint surfaces to slide back and forth with very little friction.

As I said, more than just a cushion pad in joints and spinal discs, the cartilage is a living tissue of cells and collagen and, therefore, requires a daily supply of nutrients to help it repair constant wear and tear. Poor nutrition (promoting a deficiency of nutrients and vitamins, and the presence of free radicals and anti-nutrients) prevents the repair process from progressing normally. The collagen first becomes less structured, and later becomes abnormal and deficient in important components. This process triggers an inflammatory reaction in which injured cells pour their enzymes into the intercellular space, damaging the tissue and producing a flow of proteins, eicosanoids and inflammatory cells.

As the degeneration and inflammation progress, the proteins and fibers that make the cartilage a strong tissue begin to weaken and dissolve. This process leaves areas that are damaged, scarred, partially ulcerated and irregular like a street full of bumps and holes that needs repair. As the joint tries to work under these conditions, usage creates friction and heat, which triggers additional swelling and pain, which spreads to the tendons and ligaments.

The body responds to this cartilage breakdown by sending calcium in an attempt to fortify and stabilize the joint. Unfortunately, this natural response results in calcium deposits, which grow and become spurs. Joint stiffness and enlargement follow. The process could still be stopped and reversed, but when the causes that created it are not addressed (and the patient concedes to Celebrex, Ibuprofen, etc., a pat on the back and no further treatment), the degeneration continues and degenerative osteoarthritis ensues.

A key issue to remember is that cartilage needs nutrients to keep it healthy and strong. Nutrition plays an important role in daily cartilage repair. If the cartilage is supplied with nutrition that provides good eicosanoids, fresh antioxidants, proteins and adequate vitamins, it will remain a healthy cartilage, quick to repair itself. If the cartilage is fed with nutrition that provides bad eicosanoids, free radicals and poor vitamin content, the health of the cartilage will become compromised. Daily wear and tear that is not repaired is the first step in joint degeneration.

Joint injury: the root of the problem

Read the following section slowly, because this is where it all begins. Joint injury is related to the relationship between the mechanical "wear and tear" process and an altered metabolism of cartilage due to lesions (areas of damaged tissue). The wasting of a joint is not just a melting away of the cartilage but rather a dynamic process in which the wasting actually *creates* further abnormal metabolism. This prevents the healthy growth of the cartilage and triggers instead an active inflammatory process that results in local swelling and heat. As the pressure of poor posture or a sports injury, for example, continuously burdens a spot on the cartilage, it is accompanied by a gradual alteration of the cells and local biochemical mechanisms for the purposes of healing. Injury causes loss of tissue. As such, the local cartilage is activated so that it can begin generating more tissue to restore itself in a process called inflammation and repair.

The concept to remember is that a lesion to the cartilage is not just a simple event. Instead, a lesion triggers an inflammation response that brings cells and proteins together in an attempt to repair the damage. This is a little like what happens when you disrupt an ant heap – many ants come to investigate, attack, and repair. It all happens automatically.

The inflammation and repair process in itself is good and helpful; the problem occurs when it becomes chronic, as in arthritis, and when continuous inflammation prevents healing from taking place. In osteoarthritis, for example, the cartilage becomes soft and loses elasticity and strength. With the thinning of the cartilage, the bone ends begin to rub together, causing heat, swelling and pain. Since the ligaments do not change in length as the cartilage thins, eventually they become too long for the joint. This means that they are no longer holding the bones of the joint together as tightly as they should, which makes the joint unstable and imbalanced. This increases the amount of rubbing, which isn't supposed to be happening in the first place, between the cartilage of the two bones of the joint, further damaging the cartilage tissue while increasing the inflammatory response (which I describe in more detail in the next chapter). A vicious circle of damage-causing-more-damage begins, and joint deterioration is inevitable.

Additionally, as the cartilage and bones rub together they react to the damage by growing out the sides of the joint; the cartilage becomes denser and the bones can develop protrusions or spurs where the ligaments attach. This is the cascade of degeneration: a complex process of cartilage wasting, inflammation, and abnormal cell growth (in the form of lumpy fibers mixed with calcium) that slowly enlarges the joints. In this progressive process of deterioration, the joint becomes oversized and bulbous.

Joint and cartilage in trouble

In a healthy joint, cartilage, ligaments and tendons work together to shield the joint against friction and impact; daily wear and tear is minimal and local tissue repair is successful. However, if part of the joint or the spine is not healthy (due to injury, bad posture, toxins, trauma, nutritional deficiency, accidents, or damage caused by free radicals, stressful physical activities, food allergies, or a poor diet) daily repair will not be successful. The small "micro" damages will not be fixed for the next day's use, and inflammation persists. When joints or the spine are used without being fully repaired, further damage occurs: the cartilage thins and erodes, muscles go into spasm, ligaments swell and pain begins (or continues). If daily activities force the area to work, the damage gets worse. Friction creates more heat, which creates more injury, and the inflammatory process is accelerated. A vicious circle begins, creating more and more pain and spasm in local muscles, which in turn creates tightness and restriction in movement and further tissue damage. The cartilage becomes trapped in a cycle of inflammation-causing damage and damage-causing inflammation.

Whether the process begins as a slow degeneration of cartilage and extends to tendons, muscles and ligaments, or it starts as tendonitis or ligament injury and moves to the cartilage, the result is similar:

pain, swelling and cartilage disease. Continuous inflammation leads to degenerative joint disease (osteoarthritis).

The inflammation triggered by this process is a complex cellular and biochemical reaction, which is explained in detail in the next chapter. If the cause that precipitated the inflammation is eliminated and the cartilage is healthy, proteins, eicosanoids and cells will work together to fix the damage. However, if the agent that caused the injury is still present, if the injury recurs, or if the cartilage is not healthy (perhaps because the person is not healthy), the inflammatory process will continue. Dysfunctional repair and degeneration ensues, which institutes the development and progression of osteoarthritis.

Repair

If the injuries are small and far apart and the healing process is adequate, there will be no progression into osteoarthritis. Successful repair will prevent it. However, if the injuries are too severe or frequent – such as with a tennis player, hard labor worker or a basketball player – the repair process may not be quick enough to prepare the joint for the next activity and repair will not be successful. On other occasions, the injury may be small but the repair process is defective, pushing the joint into osteoarthritis. In fact, regardless of whether the injury is small or large, the repair process is the main factor in the healing of the joint and the prevention of arthritis. Let me rephrase this extremely important concept: whether the joint will heal or will develop arthritis depends on the repair process. Explaining the causes of a defective repair process is one of the primary aims of this book.

> Whether a joint will heal or will be pushed into arthritis depends on the efficiency of the body's natural repair process.

Sorry, but there was no way to make the last few pages any simpler. We've been dealing with a very complex mechanism that you need to grasp if you want to understand why integrative medicine works. If there is something you don't understand, or you want to read more about the subject, you can fax me your questions at (561) 744-5349, or e-mail them to Igal50@aol.com, or send them by regular mail to the address shown on my website (www.jupiterinstitute.com).

> Arthritis is not just a passive erosion of the joint, but an active process of inflammation, degeneration and unsuccessful repair.

At this time, it is important to understand the following sentence for the management of arthritis: Arthritis is not just a passive erosion of the joint, but an active process of inflammation, degeneration and unsuccessful repair.

We need to comprehend that the inflammatory-degenerative process of arthritis is not like a tragedy people watch on television, to which they may say "Oh, it's awful...but there's nothing I can do." With arthritis, there is something that sufferers can do, but they must assume the responsibility of doing it. Of course, they can shield themselves behind the excuse that it is too difficult to understand, or too complicated. Well... yes, it's a bit complicated, I agree. But what's the alternative? To keep taking pills until the day the orthopedic surgeon is standing over you with a scalpel?

Once the complex process of arthritis is understood, it will be clear that taking anti-inflammatory pills will not fix it. A comprehensive management regimen such as the one offered by the Jupiter Institute Pain Program is able to treat the intimate mechanism of arthritis and provide a beneficial effect in addressing the root causes of the arthritic condition. I invite both patients and doctors to engage in similar approaches in order to combat this disabling disease.

Using the seven points of our program, a significant improvement and even a reversal of the arthritis process can be achieved. Studies show that adopting a diet like our Jupiter Institute Omega Diet can have a favorable effect in healing the degenerative and inflammatory processes of arthritis and injuries. This favorable effect can be enhanced with certain supplements and vitamins. Research also shows that both chiropractic and acupuncture treatments have a positive effect in healing painful joints and injuries, and many books have been published showing how certain exercises and physical therapy aid in the repair process of the ailing tissues. But when all these therapies are combined and integrated, the sum of the whole is a lot more powerful than any of the individual components by themselves. The beneficial effects are tremendous, and the impact in decreasing symptoms and improving the quality of life is enormous.

CHAPTER THREE

Understanding Inflammation

The four classic signs

 When Bertha made her first visit to my clinic, she was 40 pounds overweight and experiencing arthritis in all her joints, extreme fatigue, chronic headaches, swelling in her legs, and respiratory allergies. This 65-year-old secretary had seen at least half of a dozen physicians. Between them, they had prescribed eight medications ranging from muscle relaxants and anti-inflammatories to anti-depressants. Yet, all of her symptoms had worsened: She was in constant pain, and she was losing her ability to earn a living.

Bertha's symptoms were classic signs of acute inflammation distinguished by the four most common indicators – heat, swelling, redness and pain. Her respiratory allergies signaled still another red flag for inflammation. Symptoms of inflammation in the body can be triggered by infection, injury, toxins and even parasites. Each cause may provoke a different set of reactions in the body, but essentially all of the reactions are similar and involve the attacking agent, the suffering local cells, and the local response of proteins,

white blood cells, and molecules called prostaglandins or eicosanoids. The battle between these three players within Bertha's body had triggered her symptoms.

To relieve Bertha's pain, stiffness, and swelling symptoms, I immediately started her on an anti-inflammatory diet. Most people find it hard to believe that diet is so important to pain relief, and Bertha was no exception. I had to convince her that she should give my diet plan an opportunity to work. Her normal dietary habits were particularly unhealthy because she was eating too much of the wrong kinds of food in an attempt to diminish her pain and anxiety. I prescribed a diet without dairy products and meat (except oily fish), taught her some basic cooking tips, then made her promise to go to the market for fresh produce every day. I also asked her to eliminate all alcohol from her life except for red wine.

Within four months of sticking to this anti-inflammatory diet, Bertha had lost 24 pounds, her headaches were less frequent, the asthma was gone, her inflammation had been reduced, and she had eliminated many of her medications. At this point, I put her on vitamin therapy and prescribed sessions with our chiropractor and our acupuncturist. After several more months, she had dropped more pounds, approaching a normal weight for her height. Most of Bertha's stiffness and pain had gone, and her flexibility had returned.

Bertha had dramatically changed both her body and her life for the better. Out of appreciation, she brought us a bottle of wine as a gift. She had reclaimed a normal life. When she tried to say thank you, she choked up with emotion. That is always the greatest gift of all for us, when our patients express their overwhelming joy and gratitude for having conquered a debilitating condition.

A Complex Process

The complex process of inflammation is the cause of degenerative arthritis and the target of our Jupiter Institute Pain Program. As painful and disabling as it may be, inflammation is the body's response to injury and infection. It is a natural, automatic process that is essential to survival, and while we cannot control the process of inflammation, we are able to exercise some influence over it.

Every human being needs a properly functioning inflammatory process to survive the many assaults from the environment. Unfortunately, on occasion this response may be exaggerated and sustained for no apparent or beneficial reason.

When an injury (physical, infectious or mechanical) occurs, inflammation is the first response. The injury triggers a chemical reaction in the body. The body, recognizing the danger, dispatches different types of cells to the affected area. These cells and chemicals are key players in the process of inflammation (and subsequent healing). Incoming cells interact with local cells, proteins and molecules in a complex reaction of defense. The aggressor, whatever it is, is attacked by molecules and "angry" cells. To picture this battle, imagine a beetle suddenly entering an anthill. Its invasion triggers a sudden burst of activity in the ant community. Some attack the invader, others repair the damage to the anthill, some observe and communicate, but all are focused on the common goal – to kill the aggressor and repair the damage.

Inflammation is far more than just a local swelling; it is the location of the extremely complex biological activity where incoming white blood cells surround invading organisms and injured cells and attempt to destroy them. It is also an area where repair-promoting molecules that are destined to reduce inflammation interact with the opposing attack-molecules that create inflammation. Both are necessary for the healing process.

In general, these molecules are called *prostaglandins,* or *eicosanoids*. They are released by local cells as well as incoming white blood cells. We refer to them as "good" or "bad," depending on whether they are promoting repair or inflammation. From here forward we will call them "good eicosanoids" (pro-repair) and "bad eicosanoids" (pro-inflammation).

THE BEGINNING

Reviewing the process of inflammation will help you understand how medications, nutrition and therapies are able to affect its mechanisms.

An initial injury starts the process of inflammation. The injury can be an intense mechanical force on an otherwise healthy cartilage or ligament, such as a football injury in a healthy 25-year-old. Or, it can be a minimal injury in an already debilitated joint, such as when a sedentary obese person climbs the stairs. Whatever the initiating event, the injured cells start to pour enzymes into the surrounding tissues. If the injury has damaged the cartilage or ligament of a joint, the enzymes will irritate the healthy cells of the joint and cause them to break down, which sets in motion a sequence of events that lead to joint inflammation (arthritis).

Once the inflammatory process starts in the joint, local proteins block the formation of new fresh cartilage. So, there is more destruction than reconstruction of the cartilage. This effect perpetuates the damage.

Scientists and doctors do not currently understand why the repair is blocked. But we do know that once the inflammatory process has started in the cartilage, it will progress unless something radical is done to shift the trend. This early sequence of damage, inflammation and repair brought to a standstill is the beginning of osteoarthritis. To review: as the enzymes trigger the inflammatory response, the area begins to swell. This is accompanied by an increase in local temperature; both events are quite obvious to the person. White blood cells arrive at the injury zone to investigate the "invader." They add some of their own enzymes into the mix, worsening the inflammatory response. At this time, the inflamed cells involved in the conflict start to produce eicosanoids, which are local molecules that interact with the cells and proteins. By this time, the injury zone looks microscopically like our anthill that has been invaded by an outside force. The incident triggers the invasion of numerous "players" – molecules that swarm around and perform different functions.

THE ROLE OF OMEGA FATTY ACIDS IN INFLAMMATION

Omega-6 and omega-3 fatty acids play a major role in the inflammatory response; they are used by the cells to produce eicosanoids. The omega-6 eicosanoids produce a strong inflammatory response, promoting swelling and hindering repair. The omega-3 eicosanoids promote anti-inflammation, encourage the decrease in swelling and push for repair. However, if omega-6 eicosanoids predominate, then the inflammatory response can be overwhelming.

Aspirin and anti-inflammatory drugs reduce inflammation and pain in the arthritic joint by intervening in this process; they block the enzymes that make omega-6 eicosanoids, while favoring omega-3 eicosanoids. As I mentioned earlier, because of the risks associated with long-term use, these drugs should only be used for a short course while the necessary lifestyle changes are implemented. These medications are discussed further in Chapter 6.

THE EICOSANOID BALANCE

Every tissue in the body – cartilage, bone, ligament, arteries, the heart and other internal organs – contains eicosanoids. They are complex molecules that coordinate the tissue's metabolic function, interacting with hormones, water, sugar, minerals and nutrients to assure proper function, adequate energy supply and waste elimination. They are very important to good health.

They are like super hormones, controlling every vital biological function of the body. When a healthy person eats well and has good metabolism, eicosanoids exhibit "good behavior" in the tissues. Because eicosanoids are the regulators of cellular function, this good behavior helps tissues work well, repair themselves and fix the daily wear and tear.

However, if a person is not healthy or has poor dietary habits, has a hormonal imbalance, is obese or diabetic, is under stress, or abuses alcohol or caffeine, eicosanoids will "behave badly" in the tissues and organs. This bad behavior causes cell damage, interferes with repair, causes inflammation and hurts the local tissues. This gives rise to multiple problems in the body. Symptoms (which vary according to the location of the bad eicosanoids) are usually slow at the onset and do not give the person any clue of what is going on. It may take years for someone to find out that their joints or arteries are ill.

Healthy people have a proper balance of good and bad eicosanoids. This creates harmony in the body as a whole, even if their functions antagonize one another. Bodily functions work well and people feel comfortable. However, numerous agents in diet and the environment are capable of breaking this healthy balance by increasing the amount of bad eicosanoids. When this happens, disease occurs, which adversely affects the organs and tissues of the body.

Omega-6, a fatty acid present in meat, dairy products, fried food and fast food – key components of the typical American diet – stimulates the production of bad eicosanoids, which upsets the good-bad eicosanoid balance. A diet containing excessive omega-6 is bad for your health; it creates an imbalance that promotes inflammation, heart disease, osteoarthritis, diabetes, strokes and even cancer.

Omega-3 fatty acid, however, generates good eicosanoids, promotes healing, favors repair and decreases inflammation and pain.

Foods containing omega-3 are good for the body; they counteract the bad effects of omega-6 fatty acids, mitigating all the adverse effects described above. In this process they are actively preventing heart disease, improving function of the brain, immune system and bowels, decreasing fatigue, headaches, arthritis and even lowering the risk of cancer. Chapter 7 shows you how to avoid foods containing omega-6, and how to increase your intake of omega-3 fatty acids.

FATS, OILS AND THE PRODUCTION OF EICOSANOIDS

There are many types of dietary fat, and many ways of classifying them: animal fats, vegetable fats, fried fats, cooked fats, man-made fats, hydrogenated fats, saturated and unsaturated fats, processed fats, trans fats, and so on. It's easy to be confused by all these designations, and difficult to remember which are good for you and which are not. In this book for simplicity's sake, I am dividing fats and oils into two categories: those that provide omega-3 fats (or omega-3 fatty acid) and those that provide omega-6 fats (omega-6 fatty acid).

To reiterate, omega-3 fats are good for health, generating good eicosanoids, while excessive amounts of omega-6 fats are detrimental to health. As you will see, however, it is the ratio between omega-6s and omega-3s in each oil that determines its overall effect in the body. Even still, it is best to limit our intake of oils, as *all* oils are high in calories.

In term of eicosanoids, our cells actually make them from the omega-3s and omega-6s that you have. Once manufactured, they migrate outside their "home" cells and interact with local cells. Eicosanoids are very local: they do not travel around but rather stay in the area where they were made, controlling the local metabolism, the flow of glucose and minerals, energy and temperature, waste disposal, water flow and other functions.

They act like the manager of a large condominium building who controls the water, electricity, air conditioning and waste disposal of every apartment. If the manager does his job well, tenants will be happy; if not, everybody suffers.

WHAT EICOSANOIDS DO AND WHERE

Eicosanoids, good and bad, work in every tissue of our body but have opposite effects.

1. **Effects on insulin.** Good eicosanoids decrease the need for insulin, improve insulin function and lower blood-sugar levels. Bad eicosanoids do the opposite; they promote diabetic conditions in the body.

2. **Effects on the cardiovascular and circulatory systems.** Good eicosanoids improve heart rhythm, decrease the pain of angina, keep arteries open and leave the platelets less sticky. Bad eicosanoids do the opposite: they make the platelets stickier, contract the arteries and increase the likelihood of angina and heart attacks.

   Bad eicosanoids cause small areas of inflammation inside the arterial walls, making the buildup of cholesterol and calcium possible, as well as the formation of arteriosclerosis or atherosclerosis (hardening of the arteries). The growth of atherosclerotic plaque impairs blood flow and obstructs the arteries and is a key factor in heart attacks and stroke. Good eicosanoids, however, keep the arteries and other blood vessels clean and their walls smooth. This prevents the formation of those micro-spots of inflammation that lead to arteriosclerosis, thus reducing the likelihood of cardiovascular disease.

3. **Effects on the brain.** Bad eicosanoids worsen anxiety and depression and disrupt brain function and cognitive abilities. Good eicosanoids, however, improve both depression and anxiety, promote tranquility, and improve mood and mental function. They also decrease the frequency and intensity of headaches and migraines.

4. **Effects on the immune system.** Good eicosanoids improve the immune system and help the body prevent diseases. Bad eicosanoids hurt the immune system, making it more difficult to prevent and recover from illness and disease.

5. **Effects on cholesterol metabolism.** Good eicosanoids increase HDL (good cholesterol) and lower triglycerides levels. A diet promoting good eicosanoids also decreases LDL (bad cholesterol) substantially. This combined effect of increasing HDL and decreasing LDL lowers the risk ratio of cholesterol, decreases arteriosclerosis and helps prevent heart attacks and strokes. This is one of the reasons why a "Mediterranean Diet" – rich in omega-3, low in omega-6 – prolongs life. Bad eicosanoids, however, do just the opposite.

6. **Effects on joints.** In joints, bad eicosanoids promote cell disruption and inflammation, interfering with the healing of daily wear and tear. They also interfere with the rebuilding of cartilage, a major cause of pain and stiffness with arthritis. Good eicosanoids, to the contrary, are healers. They rebuild cartilage, help the injured areas and prevent the formation of arthritis.

7. **Effects on the gastrointestinal system.** Bad eicosanoids irritate the bowels and interfere with their function, triggering constipation and colitis. Good eicosanoids promote the secretion of mucus that coats the inside of the stomach and protects against acidity in the digestive system. By the way, this is how anti-inflammatory medications cause stomach irritation. They stimulate bad eicosanoids in the stomach, which decreases the secretion of protective mucus, causing stomach irritation and even ulcers.

8. **Effects on the lungs.** Certain types of bad eicosanoids, called leukotrienes, worsen asthma. Leukotrienes arrive with the white blood cells and produce inflammation of the bronchi, contraction of the entire airway, and the secretion of mucus, obstructing the

passage of air. This causes wheezing and shortness of breath. The same process of swelling, congestion and secretion occurs in the nose (rhinitis, allergic rhinitis). Steroids such as cortisone and a medication, Singulair, improve the symptoms of asthma and rhinitis by blocking the leukotrienes. However, care must be taken to use these only when necessary, and only until proper lifestyle changes, including dietary, can be made.

9. **Effect on the body as a whole.** In general, eicosanoids affect the whole body. Good eicosanoids decrease fatigue, body ache, stiffness and pain. Bad eicosanoids, on the contrary, cause fatigue and increase body aches that trigger a worsening of pain while promoting water retention and swelling in the body. They make fibromyalgia worse.

10. **Effects on the genitourinary system.** Good eicosanoids ease symptoms of menopause and PMS in women and improve erection in men.

11. **Effects on the skin.** Good eicosanoids decrease hair loss, help the skin recover from acne and improve eczema, dry skin, cracked skin, itch and dandruff.

12. **Other effects.** Good eicosanoids decrease chronic fatigue and have an anti-cancer effect.

You should now have a good idea of how good eicosanoids keep you well and how bad eicosanoids make your life miserable.

FREE RADICALS AND ANTIOXIDANTS

Free radicals are molecules generated by the metabolic processes of the body. In normal situations, our bodies use free radicals in specific chemical reactions like glucose metabolism and processing fatty acid. When there is an overabundance of free radicals, however, tissue damage occurs. In excess, free radicals attack cells and other molecules by breaking them apart and stealing electrons; the result is called *oxidation*, which you can think of as something similar to an accelerated rusting process when metal is exposed to water and air. We can compare free radicals with using bleach to remove stains in clothing: as long as we use it correctly it will be effective, but if too much is used it will cause damage to the surrounding areas.

Injuries and inflammation disrupt local metabolic pathways and cause a leakage of free radicals that damages the surroundings like a leaking bottle of bleach. Excess of free radicals may also be caused by poor food choices (fried foods, excessive animal products, excessive alcohol), smoking and exposure to chemicals, or be triggered by stress, diabetes or other diseases.

The presence of free radicals in an area of injury or inflammation cause the inflammatory process to be more damaging and longer lasting. Free radicals also destroy omega-3s, attacking and oxidizing them, which prevents them from generating the good eicosanoids needed for repair. If your body is full of free radicals, the good effects of omega-3 in your diet will be neutralized. Free radicals are definitely "bad guys" in the context of inflammation.

As we said, free radicals are produced in abundance through poor dietary habits, smoking, alcohol and drug abuse (including the overuse of pharmaceutical drugs), uncontrolled stress, obesity or diabetes. They are also in excess when a disease is not well-treated (dental infection, chronic bronchitis, liver conditions, etc). Additionally, if a person's primary diet is comprised primarily of fast food, fried and processed food, and foods with high amounts of fat and sugar, they will have an overabundance of omega-6. Omega-6, you may recall, produces an excess of pro-inflammatory bad eicosanoids that also neutralize the pro-repair good eicosanoids that come from omega-3.

People who fall into this category are in what we can call an *omega-6/bad eicosanoid/free-radical state*. They become ill more easily; they have more illness and disease; injuries and inflammations take longer to heal; their diseases are more intense and lengthy; and they will be prescribed more medications to address the numerous symptoms related to their ill health. Moreover, their immune systems, already in a weakened state, will become even more so. This puts them at a higher risk not only for developing the diseases mentioned above, but becoming disabled by them and experiencing an early and potentially painful death.

People who live in this state will get into trouble sooner or later. Since their disease develops slowly – sometimes very slowly – these people will not see symptoms until the disease is much advanced. At this point, the damage to the tissue and the organs has been done. Some find out about their joint situation, for example, when they are already full of arthritis. Others find out about coronary artery blockages when they get a heart attack. Still others suffer from fatigue, headache or bowel problems without even knowing that their bodies are sick. Some get diabetes and cancer. But most refuse to accept the idea that nutrition and lifestyle has a lot to do with the onset of these diseases, and some will never know what actually killed them.

Here's something to remember: bad food kills slowly, and it is a major cause of *every* disease of inflammation.

Good food, on the other hand, which contains helpful nutrients like *antioxidants* that neutralize free radicals, promotes the proper assimilation of omega-3s for the production of good eicosanoids. Antioxidants work against (*anti*) oxidation and protect omega-3s from being attacked by free radicals.

People who live in what we call *omega-3/good eicosanoid/ antioxidant state* will enjoy an abundance of the good, healing eicosanoids. They will be rewarded with faster healing and better health. Additionally, the onset of many diseases will be delayed or prevented altogether.

To reach this state, it is not necessary to eat solely omega-3 foods. Just eat more of them while consuming fewer omega-6 foods. Approximately 5% of the average American diet is omega-3, which is quite low. Many millions of Americans don't even achieve that percentage, which results in a very poor omega-6/omega-3 ratio of approximately 20-to-30:1. This is in stark contrast to the ideal ratio of omega-3s to omega-6s of 3-4:1. To reach this omega-3 state, most people need to increase their omega-3 intake by 25-30% while substantially decreasing their intake of omega-6s.

Diets such as our Jupiter Institute Omega Diet, described in Chapter 7, help people withdraw from the omega-6/bad eicosanoid/ free-radical state and achieve the omega-3/good eicosanoid/ antioxidant state. The transition to an omega-3/good eicosanoid/ antioxidant state decreases inflammation and damage, and provides the internal environment necessary for healing and repair. Let me emphasize that for anyone struggling with pain, arthritis or injuries, the beneficial effects of this diet are greatly reinforced and enhanced by participation in regular, appropriate exercise, and a positive combination of chiropractic care, acupuncture treatments and physical therapy. Again, an integrative approach such as our seven-point program outlined in Chapter 1 is the best way to treat conditions such as osteoarthritis.

CHAPTER FOUR

A Battle Plan for Neck and Back Pain

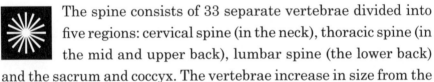 The spine consists of 33 separate vertebrae divided into five regions: cervical spine (in the neck), thoracic spine (in the mid and upper back), lumbar spine (the lower back) and the sacrum and coccyx. The vertebrae increase in size from the cervical area to the lumbar area in accordance with the amount of weight they need to support.

Vertebrae are separated by round cartilaginous cushions, known as discs, which are made of fibers and thick cartilage. They allow a certain degree of motion between one vertebra and the next.

Vertebrae are attached to one another by ligaments, tendons and muscles. This creates a column that is strong and flexible, and able to extend and rotate. The sides of the vertebral column have

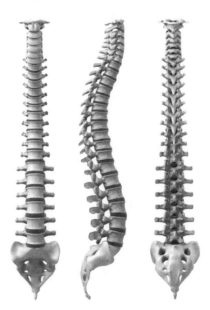

small holes, called *foramina,* through which the nerves pass. These nerves extend from the spinal cord to the outside and connect our

central nervous system to muscles, skin and organs. A single *foramen* is shaped by a notch between two vertebrae in an area exposed and in contact with the intervertebral disc. This can be a weak point for a nerve since an arthritis condition between two vertebrae or a bulging in the disc may result in irritation, pinching or squeezing of the nerve. Whether irritated or pinched, the nerve conduction is stimulated, and pain is felt. This is called *neuritic pain* or *neuralgia.* The suffering of the nerve is called *neuritis* or *neuropathy.* Therefore, you can say that sciatica is a neuritic pain caused by a neuropathy of the roots of the sciatic nerve.

Understanding some anatomy – in addition to how pain occurs – will help you see why a program such as the Jupiter Institute Pain Program can be effective.

There are many causes of pain but for the purpose of this chapter we will divide them into:

1. **Pain due to organic causes** such as kidney stones, digestive-system diseases, cardiovascular diseases, tumors, infections, etc. (I will not address this type of pain here; we would need a short textbook of medicine to do so), and:

2. **Pain caused by musculoskeletal disorders of the spine and limbs,** which we will examine in greater detail here. That is the purpose of this book.

Pain in this second category can be *acute* or *chronic.* Acute pain is essentially a new pain, one that started today or a few days ago. The pain must have commenced within 30 days to be called acute pain. If the pain lasts more than one month but less than six months, it is called sub-acute pain. Pain lasting more than six months is called chronic pain.

Depending on its severity, chronic pain can be a persistent nightmare, dominating the sufferer and causing physical, mental and emotional weakness and even depression. Chronic pain, like arthritis, needs to be understood, which means that we must look for, find and address its *root causes* in order to achieve healing. It is a multi-factorial disorder requiring the coordinated efforts of a treatment team, since the resources of a single practitioner are generally insufficient to properly identify and treat all of the involved factors. This is a critical point that needs repeating. Doctors and patients must understand and accept the fact that a solo practitioner is generally unable to address the variety of causes of chronic pain and the resulting problems and symptoms. Furthermore, only one or two treatments of a single therapeutic approach are typically unsuccessful at treating a chronic pain condition, most of which take years to develop. Chronic pain conditions require the combined efforts of a team over a period of time. Here are examples of single-therapy approaches that are typical today: A woman with neck pain takes only painkillers and anti-inflammatories; a man who has had shoulder pain for eight months receives one cortisone shot and takes Ibuprofen. These are just two examples of how treatment can be confined to symptom management, while the underlying condition worsens. In both of these cases, there is no particular broad therapeutic approach that addresses the cause of the pain or that promotes the healing and repair of the condition.

Pain means injury and injury demands repair. Repair demands a plan of treatment and not just pills. The success of any treatment plan depends on a thorough understanding of *the causes* of the pain – by both the patient and the doctor. Furthermore, *both patient and doctor must understand that the causes of chronic pain will never by addressed by a pill.* Once this understanding is firmly intact, a comprehensive approach needs to be applied and followed. Without it, healing will be unlikely. The comprehensive approach must include complementary medicine for long-term relief, and both patients and doctors must open their minds in order to embrace and use it.

Neck Pain Caused By Trauma

Fractures and dislocations of the spine must be considered first in any person with a recent history of neck pain or injury. Therefore, an X-ray of the spine is needed in every case of significant neck pain, and after an injury or accident.

A number of terms are used interchangeably to refer to the typical soft tissue injury of the neck, including "whiplash injury," "cervical sprain" and "neck sprain." In the case of neck sprain, the ligaments that hold the vertebrae together are sprained or over-stretched, often by the head snapping backwards. If the injury is severe, one vertebra may slide forward out of place and compress the spinal cord. This creates an urgent situation that requires a visit to the emergency room. However, if the sprain is mild, the person will just feel pain and stiffness in the neck area.

Whiplash injury is a severe strain of the neck caused by sudden violent movement, damaging muscles, tendons and ligaments. The spine is such a thick web of ligaments, tendons, nerves and muscular fibers that it is easy for an injury to damage all four of these structures at the same time. Imagine a sheaf of uncooked spaghetti that suffers a blow: not just one strand cracks but several, and on different levels. Similarly, whiplash may create many simultaneous micro-centers of injury.

Although job- and sports-related injuries may occasionally cause these problems, most instances of whiplash result from rear-end automobile collisions. The typical injury occurs as the head is first flexed and then forcibly overextended beyond its normal range of motion.

Significant injuries will affect not only muscles, ligaments and tendons but also the joints and cartilage of the spine, as well as the nerve roots. There are multiple types of injuries including sudden elongation of nerves and ligaments, muscle tears, ligament sprains and cartilage and tendon injuries.

Although one particular muscle or ligament may take the brunt of the damage, typically many very small areas of injury result.

Since cells are torn and damaged, each of these micro-injuries triggers the inflammatory process. Just like when an egg is cracked and the egg white leaks through the crack, torn and damaged cells leak their inside protoplasm and enzymes, which scatter among the surrounding cells. This process ends up damaging neighboring cells. In a slow and continuous chain of events, cells that were first damaged die and those that were unhurt begin to sustain damage. Those cells eventually die, freeing their protoplasm and enzymes, and hurting more cells in addition to previously unharmed cells. The destruction spreads and increasing numbers of cells become injured and die. This process generates tissue irritation (inflammation). As the inflammatory process progresses, it extends over a larger area, worsening the swelling and progressively increasing the heat and pain.

Local irritation and tissue damage can also cause muscle spasms. When this happens, blood flow is reduced, causing even more suffering among the cells. The intense inflammatory process continues, triggering the production of eicosanoids in large quantity, which attracts more white blood cells. These white blood cells arrive at the inflamed area and draw in even more enzymes and eicosanoids. After several days, each one of the micro-injury areas will have transformed itself into a complex center of inflammation. This explains why sudden neck injuries caused by auto accidents, jobs, or sports activity hurt even more after a few days. The majority of conventional medical treatment involves – almost exclusively – the prescription of muscle relaxants and pain relievers. While these pharmaceuticals may result in the temporary remediation of symptoms, they do not address the underlying causes of ongoing inflammation and, therefore, cannot heal the injury. Most injuries trigger a complex biological and physiological response that requires a multi-disciplinary approach. Anti-inflammatory nutrition, chiropractic care, physical therapy and other forms of alternative treatments work synergistically to eliminate underlying inflammation in the body – and in the micro-center of the injury – which allows for permanent healing.

Reviewing the relationship between anatomy and the pain process will help you understand the value of the treatment plan described at the end of this chapter.

Neck Pain Not Due To Trauma

The cervical spine – the spine in the neck area – is unique. It has a motion capacity unlike any other part of the spine. It can flex and extend, rotate and bend to the sides. Thanks to this mobility it also has a unique exposure to all types of injuries caused by falls, sports, work-related accidents and poor posture.

Many of these injuries result in micro-injuries in the ligaments, joints and cartilage of the spine, which accumulate over time. After many years of silent progression, these lesions slowly cause the discs to flatten and bulge. The ligaments give way, tear and calcify, and the cartilage of the joints deteriorates. This is a process called *degenerative disc disease,* and it may remain silent without symptoms for many years. However, as the condition progresses, a trigger event finally occurs bringing attention to the weakness. The trigger events can be a fall, an accident, a job-related injury, poor posture, sleeping on the couch, whiplash, or other physical strains. The inflammation caused by this event ends the silent period of this process by activating the symptoms of pain, stiffness and decreased mobility. Because the cervical spine contains a tight bundle of nerves, the pain caused by the degenerative disc disease may be felt in the neck, but may also radiate to the shoulders, arm and even to the hands.

On many occasions, the alarming symptom is not the pain but rather the tingling, numbness and even weakness of the arm. Whatever the symptoms are and whatever the cause that triggered them, the initial steps in management are an evaluation by the doctor, and the review of the X-rays of the cervical spine. Then – and only then – a treatment program can be decided. Treatment options may include medications, physical therapy, traction, injections, integrative medicine, massage, exercise or a consultation with a specialist. Part of the evaluation may include an MRI exam and measuring of nerve conduction velocities.

As the treatment modality is decided, patient and physicians must be aware of two things. First, there is an old degenerative process, which means that a complete return to normal is not possible. Second, there is an ongoing inflammatory process in the spine, which means there are areas of swelling, cell injury, eicosanoid activity and heat. Since the degree of inflammation and cell injury varies from case to case, treatments vary as well. One thing is for sure: an anti-inflammatory program, with anti-inflammatory medication and an anti-inflammatory diet, is essential if one wants to focus on tissue repair and not just masking the symptoms.

Neck pain can be the result of four main causes:

a. a **traumatic injury,** such as in a whiplash or fall, **in an otherwise healthy neck.**

b. a **traumatic injury in the neck that may already be affected by a degenerative arthritic process.** (This explains why sometimes a small injury can cause such a storm of pain and disability.)

c. a **non-traumatic injury** that has been evolving for a long time and finally starts to produce symptoms (and pain or tingling starts for no apparent cause). It may be scoliosis of the spine or an extremely slow, progressive bulging disc.

d. **a non-arthritic and non-traumatic condition,** such as a cyst, tumor or neuropathy, etc., affecting the neck or its structures.

The first step in evaluating the cause of neck pain, therefore, is to see a doctor for an X-ray of the neck to rule out cause (a), and to make sure that it is an injury and not an arthritis-related problem.

An X-ray will also help to determine whether the problem is indeed (a), (b) or (c). The X-ray findings will determine the treatment. Additional evaluation includes an MRI, complete blood tests, and possibly even a second opinion from a consultant.

So far so good. However, if the distress is caused by (b) or (c), there is likely an old and/or new injury process occurring in the cervical spine, which also means that there is an active inflammatory process in one or more locations in the spine. There could be more or less pain, and there could be more or less degeneration or bulging of the discs. But, for sure, there is an inflammatory process somewhere in the spine.

From our previous discussion, we know that at the center of these inflammatory pockets cells are being injured and are pouring their enzymes onto surrounding cells. Eicosanoids are interacting with proteins and cells; there is swelling and heat, there are numerous white blood cells and waste products, and cartilage is being eroded because its fibers are disintegrating. If you could look at the process under a microscope, it is like the disrupted anthill that I mentioned earlier, teeming with ants frantically moving everywhere.

The purpose of the inflammation is twofold: as a defense against further injury, and as a reconstructive force for the injured area. Inflammatory cells, proteins, enzymes and eicosanoids all interact in the process. The eicosanoids, which are produced by cells from omega fatty acids, can be of the good type or the bad type. As described in the previous chapter, the good eicosanoids will try to decrease inflammation and promote repair while the bad type will do the opposite. The ratio of good to bad eicosanoids will depend on the magnitude of the injury, the state of health of the tissues, and the nutritional value of the foods consumed by the person.

Whatever treatment is chosen, it must take into account *both* the cause of the injury as well as this inflammatory process. This is a critical point. If the pain and disability are just treated with pills, or with pills and massage, then the root cause of the problem is not being treated. When the real cause of the problem is neglected, and the symptoms are masked with pills, the problem continues to grow and worsens with time. Those who suffer from injuries or arthritic conditions in the neck should not rely on pills for treatment. It is acceptable to take medications for a short period of time; however, this should not be the main and only therapy utilized for healing, but rather part of the global treatment plan.

Again, the main treatment should target the cause of the problem *and* the inflammatory process. The cause of the problem can be treated with physical therapy, traction, manipulation, massage, a cervical collar, special pillow, injections, chiropractic manipulations, exercise, etc. The inflammatory process should be treated with an anti-inflammatory program that includes a short course of anti-inflammatory medication, an anti-inflammatory diet, and supplements, including omega-3s and antioxidants, known to be powerful anti-inflammatory agents.

Let me elaborate. The idea that we can fight inflammation by just taking anti-inflammatories and/or cortisone (Prednisone, Medrol, etc.) is an outdated concept. Just as penicillin was used when it was initially discovered for every bacterial infection, nowadays we know better, and have different options. So, now that we understand the entire inflammatory and injury process much better, we must modernize and update our treatment programs so that the painful conditions that afflict people can actually be eradicated.

LOW BACK PAIN

Low back pain is a frequent complaint and may be localized above the buttock area or on the buttocks. It is generally intense, affecting one side more than the other. The pain may radiate down the thigh or leg (when it is known as sciatica), indicating that one or more nerve roots are being pinched. The cause, most likely, would be the same as that triggering the back pain.

Like any arthritic condition, low back pain may be activated by general disease or by a local cause. Numerous general diseases and metabolic disorders can affect the lower back, along with localized spinal disorders, ranging from cysts and tumors to fractures and genetic disorders. Most of the local causes are related to acute ligament sprain and muscular strain, or acute worsening of an old disc problem. Hence, the first step in the management of low back pain is an evaluation by a medical doctor.

The second step is to decide whether blood tests are needed, which should occur when there is suspicion of a generalized metabolic or rheumatologic condition such as anemia, lupus, rheumatoid arthritis, or infection, for example. The third step is an X-ray of the lumbar spine and, on occasion, an X-ray of the pelvic bone as well. In dynamic medical offices, with physicians attentive to the patients' concerns, blood test and X-ray results may be obtained within 48 to 72 hours – or less – and a determination can be made about the cause and treatment of the problem.

Major diseases need to be ruled out first. These include tumors, cancers, metabolic diseases, congenital disorders, severe osteoporosis, Paget's disease, rheumatoid arthritis, old fractures, pelvic disorders, kidney diseases, vascular disorders and other conditions.

If all of these diseases have been ruled out, the focus will be on the spine and related areas. If the findings in the X-ray suggest spine and vertebral disease, treatment can be initiated according to the symptoms of the patient and the X-ray findings.

A CAT scan or an MRI is not routinely necessary. Whether they are advised depends on the doctor's evaluation. The most frequent cause of low back pain is what is known as a bulging disc, or degenerative disc disease. In most cases the problem has been brewing for years, with slow protrusion or *herniation* of the disc into the spinal canal, with slow displacement of the vertebrae to the front or to the back, or with the slow progression of scoliosis. Other slow-motion events that have taken years to deform the problem area include calcification of ligaments, mechanical nerve root compression, flattening of the discs, traumatic tissue breakdown, loss of mobility between the vertebrae, and degenerative arthritis of the different parts of the vertebral joint.

All of these conditions are the result of multiple areas of micro-injuries and lesions due to heavy lifting, falls, accidents, poor posture, sports or work-related stress. The effect of these injuries and lesions accumulate through the years; gravity and body weight also aggravate the situation.

Eventually, one of two things happens. Either a trivial event (such as standing up, sitting down, bending over or taking a short walk) triggers severe back pain, or a fall, accident, sports injury or job-related injury triggers a cascade of events: pains, spasm, inflammation, heat and gait disorder.

In either one of these scenarios, a new disc herniation (bulging) with new inflammation has been added to an old chronic process. While the disc herniation causes mechanical compression of the nerves and tissues, the new inflammation brings swelling, cellular disruption, enzymes and eicosanoids. Good and bad eicosanoids will be present but in a ratio that depends, among other things, on the magnitude of the injury, the state of health of the person and their nutrition.

This picture varies from case to case. In some people, there is more inflammation and less herniation. Others show a large herniation of the disc but only a small amount of inflammation. In either case, treatment has to focus on the two main processes: herniation and inflammation. Hence, some part of treatment should be concentrated on relieving the bulging while other parts of treatment should focus on relieving the inflammation. Simply taking anti-inflammatories and pain medications will provide no healing and may mask a serious problem. Remember, while pills relieve the symptoms of the problem, the real cause of the problem is not being addressed, so the actual condition is likely to worsen with time.

Neck and back disorders may have different symptoms, but they have one thing in common: the presence of injury and inflammation. The inflammatory process, described in detail in Chapter 3, is usually characterized by a cascade of broken cells, scattered enzymes, good and bad eicosanoids and repair cells, and is accompanied by swelling and heat. The inflammation present in each one of these lesions shares responsibility for the pain and swelling of the problem area.

Free radicals, as we've seen before, are harmful molecules that damage the cells and prolong the healing of the injury. Antioxidants, on the other hand, are "good" molecules that neutralize free radicals. Antioxidants are, therefore, called anti-inflammatory molecules while free radicals are pro-inflammatories. Among the cells and proteins of the inflammatory cascade, eicosanoids, free radicals and antioxidants do their share in helping or disrupting the healing process.

The winner of this inflammatory battle determines whether the healing process is shortened or prolonged. Any treatment of low back pain or neck pain must take the inflammatory process into account. This will greatly influence the healing process and determine whether or not the inflammation subsides or remains.

SCIATICA AND ARM PAIN

Pain in the upper or lower limbs can be very misleading. It can be caused by an injury or disease in any part of the limb, including muscular disease, arthritis, and tendonitis or bone disease. Pain can also be caused by an irritation of the nerve that feeds the limb. In this case, even though the pain is felt in the limb, it is a radiated pain. The problem is indeed at the spine. Such is the case with shooting pains down the arm, or with an achy or numb arm. This is akin to the sciatic conditions that we discussed in the previous section, whereby pain in the leg is caused by a compression or irritation of the roots of the sciatic nerve in the area adjacent to the spine.

The pain can be constant or intermittent, sudden or progressive, sharp or dull. It is characterized by pain radiating down the arm or leg, which at times can be felt as a stabbing or an electrical sensation. The arm pain in these cases is known as a pinched nerve, *neuritis* or *neuropathy,* and its equivalent in the leg is called *sciatica.* Both represent a similar condition – an irritated nerve.

These two conditions have an inflammatory process in common at the root of the nerve. There may also be a traumatic, mechanical or metabolic condition at that level, but either way, local inflammation is present. This means that treatment should focus on relieving both the causes of the nerve irritation and the local inflammation. These conditions are triggered by bulging (herniated) discs, spinal stenosis, ligament sprain, spinal arthritis, muscular irritation, etc. Each requires a different treatment approach. The local inflammation indicates that tissue damage is in progress at the center of the problem. This process is active, with inflammatory cells, swelling, good and bad eicosanoids, heat, enzymes and attempts at repair.

As with all the painful conditions described in the previous pages, any treatment program that attempts to bring relief must consider this inflammatory process and try to heal it. You simply cannot heal a significant inflammatory process *and* a bulging disc area with pills or a little bit of physical therapy. If nothing is done for both the relief of the inflammatory process and the reduction of the bulging, there will be no real improvement.

THE BATTLE PLAN

The plan to heal all the conditions we've described in this chapter – in the neck, spine, nerves, tendons, back or muscles – is part of our Jupiter Institute Pain Program. The plan embraces prescription of anti-inflammatory medications for a short course, which we will review in Chapter 6, as well as anti-bulging weapons and an anti-inflammatory diet, which we call the Jupiter Institute Omega Diet, discussed in detail in Chapter 7.

Highlights of the Battle Plan are:

A. Anti-inflammatory weapons

1. *Anti-inflammatory medications.* See Chapter 6.

2. *Anti-inflammatory diet.* The diet is aimed at increasing the intake of anti-inflammatory omega-3 fatty acids and antioxidants while decreasing the intake of pro-inflammatory omega-6 and free radicals. See Chapter 7.

3. *Dietary supplements.* Supplements including omega-3, omega-9, antioxidants and vitamins, all known to have a powerful anti-inflammatory effect.

B. Anti-bulging weapons

1. *Chiropractor manipulation.* No other profession will provide such a beneficial effect in reducing the mechanical effect of a herniated disc.

2. *Physical therapy.* Not just any physical therapy, but rather a treatment protocol administered by a therapist who follows the instructions of a chiropractor, who also knows what they are doing. It is best to have a skilled chiropractor and physical therapist working together as a team.

3. *Exercises.* These should be supervised by both the chiropractor and the physical therapist. See Chapter 10.

All these treatments are complemented by acupuncture, a natural modality that heals the injured area in a physiological and energetic way. This is the path to real healing. It is the course we follow in our Jupiter Institute Pain Program, and the one that we encourage both patients and doctors to adopt. I urge you to design a similar program for yourself if there is no team currently available in the area where you live. If you have questions on how to do this, fax me your request at (561) 744-5349 or e-mail your question to (Igal50@aol.com).

CHAPTER FIVE

Understanding Common Painful Injuries

In the aftermath of injury from a motor vehicle accident, the human body sometimes responds with a series of new health challenges. They are like a row of dominoes falling against each other, causing a sudden and rapidly advancing degenerative process. Once the chain reaction starts, it is difficult to stop the process using conventional medical therapies based on pharmaceutical drugs.

Martha was 32 years old and six months pregnant when a car accident resulted in an injury that produced neck pain at her right shoulder. She overate to try and relieve the pain and anxiety, and was soon obese. After the birth of her child, she felt so tender, swollen and achy that she could not breastfeed her baby.

With three prescriptions from a psychiatrist and more drugs from other physicians, it was no wonder that Martha developed chronic stomach upset and heartburn. Rashes appeared on her body, along with severe back pain, and numbness in her right arm. Her symptoms were multiplying and getting worse despite all of the drugs she was taking.

She came to our clinic initially for our weight loss program, but it was clear to me that we needed to treat her swelling and inflammation first. Once this was handled, we could then address the injury from her accident, which also contributed to her weight problem. It took me several days to convince her that treatment should begin with our dietary program. Then the acupuncture and chiropractic sessions to treat her injury would be more successful.

After a month on our diet program, Martha lost 18 pounds – most of that from the water retention caused by the inflammation. Her stiffness and pain decreased, and her rashes were going away. By the second month she had lost nine additional pounds, her joints no longer hurt, and she was able to discard two-thirds of her medications. At this point, we were able to begin the sessions with our chiropractor and acupuncturist to treat the neck and shoulder problems caused by the car accident.

Every vehicular accident, serious fall, or sports injury has the potential to cause a range of significant traumas to body organs and bones. With car accidents, the most common injuries that I see involve whiplash and neck sprains. The symptoms and the steps that victims go through before reaching our clinic are typically very similar.

Four professional men ranging in age from 22 to 53, all of whom had been rear-ended and suffered neck and shoulder pain, illustrate this category of distressed patients. All of them had been to orthopedic physicians and neurologists before seeing us; all had had cortisone shots and had taken anti-inflammatories, muscle relaxants and pain killers. All had numbness in their hands and forearms. All experienced headaches, fatigue, sleep deprivation and stomach problems from the pills they took, accompanied by weight gain. All begin to drink more alcohol in an attempt to numb the pain. All reported that their professional effectiveness (lawyer, banker, engineer and architect) had been compromised by their symptoms.

We treated each of them using the same regimen: an anti-inflammatory diet, and chiropractic treatments along with physical therapy and massage. On the second week, we started them on acupuncture. Within a month, every single one of them was pain free and able to function effectively in life again without drugs or alcohol.

OVERVIEW

This chapter focuses on common acute injuries, including rotator cuff injuries, sprained joints and ligaments, torn and pulled muscles, tendonitis and bursitis.

These conditions commonly share the experience of an injury with the ensuing tissue disruption, broken cells, inflammation and pain. Each of them requires prompt evaluation by a doctor – an orthopedist, an internist, a general practitioner or a chiropractor. All require some form of treatment, such as physical therapy, rest, massage, medications, manipulation or a combination. But, in addition, all these injuries require an anti-inflammatory program. Each one of these lesions (injuries) is not just an area of broken tissues but rather a small center where an inflammatory storm has begun.

Although inflammation can be decreased and controlled with anti-inflammatory medications, such as Naproxen, Motrin, Aleve, Ibuprofen, Celebrex, etc., these medications will not promote the beneficial effect of the eicosanoids in the healing process. Our purpose here is to show how a person can influence the eicosanoid system so it will assist in the healing of the injury. Once the process of inflammation is understood, people in any of these four injury groups can positively influence the healing process: they can reduce inflammation thereby promoting a faster recovery. Yes, a person has control over the repair of their injuries.

ROTATOR CUFF INJURY

The shoulder is one of the largest joints of the body and prone to many injuries. Instead of ligaments, it is held together by muscles and tendons known as the rotator cuff. Because of the lack of ligaments, any weakness in the rotator cuff muscles makes it easy for the joint to lose alignment and hurt. Injuries to the rotator cuff muscles are usually secondary to sports activities, work, falls or gardening. A rotator cuff injury can also occur when falling on the arm, lifting heavy objects, and abusing the shoulder through improper or excessive weight lifting, sport activities and repetitive manual work. When this occurs, the rotator cuff muscles become stretched, and the joint loses its alignment and squeezes the tendons, causing pain and inflammation. Typical symptoms include pain, stiffness, shoulder-arm weakness and loss of motion.

A rotator cuff tear is a more advanced injury, more painful and more disabling. It requires extra intense and prolonged therapy, and, on occasion, even surgery. When the rotator cuff is injured, as in any injury to muscles, an inflammation process starts in the area of the lesion. Hence, management should include visiting a doctor, getting an X-ray to rule out fracture, and getting physical therapy, but also paying particular attention to the inflammatory process.

The proper treatment of rotator cuff injuries that don't require surgery is a good example of integrative medicine. If the X-rays are negative, the first step is to stop all aggravating activities to that shoulder. Then continue with:

- physical therapy treatment;
- exercise instructions given by the therapist;
- prescription of anti-inflammatories;
- anti-inflammatory diet (i.e. our Jupiter Institute Omega Diet);
- chiropractic evaluation for possible manipulation to decrease muscular tension in the neck and back; *and,*
- supplements like omega-3 gel caps and antioxidants (natural healers).

On many occasions (but not all), acupuncture will expedite the healing as well. People who follow this integrative approach stand a much better chance of faster and better healing.

SPRAINED LIGAMENTS

A ligament is a bundle of fibers that goes like a bridge between the two bones of a joint, attaching and holding them together. A sprain is defined as a stretching or tearing of a ligament caused by a forced movement. When it is simple, there is a minimal disruption of the fibers of the ligament, causing swelling, pain and joint stiffness. Severe sprain may cause total rupture of the ligament with marked swelling and joint instability. Although sprains are more commonly found on the ankle, they also occur in the knee, lower back and neck.

To get the idea of a sprain, imagine a bundle of spaghetti suffering a sudden blow. Although the bundle itself may not break completely, much of the spaghetti will tear, breaking many fibers. Each one of these fibers is like a cell and the tearing will create a micro-spot of injury, which will generate a micro-spot of inflammation, swelling, heat and pain. This brings eicosanoids and white blood cells into the area. The white blood cells bring even more eicosanoids with them and the process of inflammation and repair continues.

Sprained Joints

A joint sprain is an injury to the ligaments of the joint. It happens most commonly after a sport injury or a fall. A mild or Grade 1 sprain simply stretches the ligament and causes pain and swelling. A moderate, or Grade 2 sprain, partially tears the ligaments and is much more painful and disabling. A severe, or Grade 3 sprain, is a complete rupture of the ligament and requires surgical repair.

When a jogger steps off of a curb and twists the ankle, simply stretching the ligament without tearing it, that is a mild – Grade 1 – sprain. When a soccer player is hit by a blow to the outside of the knee pushing the knee inside, the blow causes severe stretching and even rupture of the medial ligament, which is a Grade 2 or 3 sprain.

Torn And Pulled Muscles

Muscle pulls and tears commonly occur in the major muscles of the arms and legs, and they represent different degrees of the same type of lesion. The injury occurs from a sudden over-stretching of the muscle beyond its limit.

The degree of over-stretching determines whether the muscle is just pulled or actually torn. In a pulled muscle, many areas suffer cell damage and cell rupture with small areas of inflammation in multiple sections of the muscle. In a torn muscle, some areas are actually separated. The degree of separation depends on the magnitude of the injury. Inflammation will be present in each one of these areas.

Bursitis

Bursae are sac-like cavities filled with oily fluid located near the joints at sites where friction occurs. They may lie between two tendons, between a tendon and a ligament, or between the tendon and the bone. Bursae facilitate normal movement and minimize friction between the moving parts. Inflammation of these bursae, called bursitis, may happen suddenly, or over a period of time. And it hurts.

Bursitis happens frequently in the shoulder but may also occur in elbow, knee, heel and other joints. The cause of this type of bursitis is usually overuse, injury, exercise, gout, infection or local inflammation. If there is arthritis in neighboring areas, inflammation from there can spread into the bursa and cause bursitis. Symptoms of bursitis are pain, localized tenderness, stiffness and limitation of movement. Swelling and increased local temperature also occur. On occasion, bursitis may spread to tendons, and cause tendonitis.

Excessive friction plays a major role in the development and progression of bursitis, which is why it typically presents in joints and areas such as the shoulder, elbow, hip, knee and heel, which experience more force from daily activities.

Because bursitis is an inflammatory process, treatment must focus on mitigating and eliminating this inflammation. Excessive usage of the affected joints will increase friction and worsen the inflammation. Therefore, in addition to anti-inflammatory treatment, rest is essential.

TENDONITIS

When a tendon is inflamed the condition is called *tendonitis.* When this inflammation involves the tendon sheath *(synovia)* it is called *tenosynovitis.* If this occurs at the level where the tendon is passing near or over a joint, the pain and swelling may give an erroneous impression of an arthritic condition. Indeed, this disorder is called para-arthritis (para = next to) and requires a different kind of treatment. The typical causes of tendonitis and tenosynovitis are overuse, daily wear and tear, exercise, injuries and repetitive micro-traumas related to work or sports activities. Some general diseases may also cause these conditions, and require further investigation.

What all of these conditions – bursitis, tendonitis, tenosynovitis and sprains – have in common is the **inflammatory process.** In all of them there is an injury, swelling, white blood cell activity, increased temperature, cellular disruptions, pain and a repair process that has been activated. Furthermore, there is an activated eicosanoid system in all of them. Inflammation does not occur for the purposes of causing pain. Inflammation is triggered by the disruption of local tissue and is the body's attempt to heal the injury. The inflammatory process is described in detail in Chapter 3.

INDIRECT CAUSES

Arthritis, tendonitis, and bursitis may also have their origin in a different area of the body. If a person has a degenerative or inflammatory process in the spine, for example, such as a disc disease or spinal arthritis, the nerves coming out of the spine will be squeezed and become irritated. This causes irritation in the area of the body that is served by that nerve. If the area served is the surface of the upper arm, then there will likely be an abnormal sensation in that area. The sensation may be rather superficial – such as tingling or numbness of the skin – which at times may be very uncomfortable. The sensation may also be a deep ache or pain as if the muscle or the bone is hurting.

However, if the irritated nerve is connected to a muscle, the irritation is transmitted directly to that muscle, causing it to become tense. This can create problems in neighboring joints. Muscles are linked to bones by tendons. At a joint, either the muscle itself or its tendons will cross over the joint – forming a bridge – to connect to another bone. At that crossing point there is usually a little bursa to facilitate sliding and avoid friction. When a muscle is tense, it is partially contracted. This contraction causes stress in both the muscle and tendons, thereby affecting the joint area. A tense muscle may squeeze the bursa, irritating it and causing it to inflame, triggering bursitis. Simultaneously, the contracted muscle may keep the two bones of the joint pressed against one another other, rubbing under pressure with minimal movement. This hurts the cartilage and ligaments, triggering the process of arthritis. Concurrently, the muscles' tendons may be suffering from excessive and unnecessary strain from contracted muscles, causing the tendons to rub against the bone with greater friction. This generates heat and inflammation that may result in tendonitis. Hence, an irritation of the nerve may cause excessive tension in the muscles and tendons around a joint, indirectly triggering bursitis, tendonitis and arthritis.

Similar situations occur with weak muscles, which can also have an origin in an irritated spinal nerve. Muscles surrounding the joints offer double protection to a joint; they hold it together, keeping the joint stable, and they provide shock absorption. If these muscles weaken, the joint may fall out of proper alignment. Additionally, the muscles will not be helpful in the distribution of pressure when a load is received. Both situations subject the cartilage to greater impact than it is designed to handle, which is likely to accelerate the degeneration of the joint over time. Therefore, muscle weakness may play a direct role in the development and progression of arthritis. If a person has either a spinal disorder with arthritis, or a bulging disc with a nerve disorder and subsequent muscle weakness, they may develop arthritis in the knee or the elbow.

In summary, irritated nerves can hurt a joint by originating a process that renders it either too loose or too tight. This is an extremely important concept, so let me rephrase it: *Nerve irritation caused by spinal arthritis or bulging discs can create either tensed or weak muscles, either of which can be the cause of osteoarthritis.* This is how a neck problem can result in a hurting shoulder. This is how a back problem may end up hurting the hip or knee. The process is usually very slow. Many years of neck trouble may result in shoulder pain. In these cases, the neck may be symptomatic (with pain and stiffness), or relatively symptom free – perhaps exhibiting only a slight decrease in the range of motion. Other times, a person is asymptomatic (without symptoms). Then one day they develop bursitis, tendonitis or arthritis in the shoulder, which may or may not be related to a neck problem. (For example, the problem may be related to a partial tear in the rotator-cuff that, after years of suffering, finally gives way and tears.) In any case, my point is this: the symptoms may present themselves as bursitis or arthritis of the hip or shoulder, or as tendonitis in the knee, but the root of the problem may be in the spine – at the origin of the nerves that extend to the hip, shoulder or knee. An abnormality in the spine and vertebrae is then the indirect cause of the problem. This is why anyone who has pain in the shoulder or arm, or in the buttocks, hips or thighs, must have a spinal evaluation, which will require X-rays. If the spine is affected, a correlation can easily be made by tracking nerves to their corresponding body areas using an anatomy book. This may help to quickly identify the real cause of the problem, and the treatment of this cause may accelerate and improve the cure. If an issue with the spine exists but is undiscovered, treatment is likely to proceed in the area displaying symptoms without addressing the root cause of the problem. This is likely to prolong and complicate the inflammatory and degenerative process. Scar formation, calcification, stiffness, chronic pain and disability that may require excessive use of medications, physical therapy, injections, medical appointments and – in some cases – surgery may result.

The idea of an *indirect cause* may seem surprising at first. But in medicine, the cause of the pain is not always located where the pain is felt. Here are some examples. A pain in the back can be caused by a gall-bladder stone (which is in the front). A kidney stone can be felt as pain in the groin. Heart trouble can be felt as a pain in the left arm. A tumor in the spine can be felt as a weakness in the leg. These symptoms are called "radiated symptoms." In this book, in order to emphasize that they may also be part of the cause of the inflammatory and injury processes, we call them the **indirect cause** of the problem.

TREATING THE REAL CAUSE

Considering all of this information at once causes me to say this: we should maintain an open mind, recognizing that there is more than one way to approach the treatment of pain in any area of our body. We now understand that a pain in the shoulder or hip may be due to arthritis, bursitis or tendonitis. We also must realize that to have a chance of reversing a pain problem we must consider the following: the inflammatory factor and its causes, and the indirect factors that may be at play.

A hurting shoulder could be treated solely as a hurting shoulder, paying no attention to anything else. However, a hurting shoulder could also be treated as an ongoing inflammatory condition, which calls for anti-inflammatory therapies. Or, we may consider the role of an indirect factor, and evaluate the neck accordingly, obtaining X-ray images and treating the pain as the result of a possible cervical spine abnormality. Or, we could use any combination of the above.

CHOICES IN TREATMENT

Now that we understand the definition and meaning of bursitis, tendonitis, rotator cuff problems, muscle and ligament sprains and strains a little better, we can address the treatment options that we integrate into our program.

- **Conventional medicine** offers the beneficial effects of physical therapy and anti-inflammatory drugs, which together provide significant relief of the symptoms. But, there is little evidence that they really heal injured tissues on their own.

- **Alternative medicine therapies** make an important contributing impact in the healing process. Studies show that in many cases people heal better and faster when alternative medicine is added to their therapy plan. Moreover, research indicates that the majority of pain and joint degeneration problems worsen when employing the two primary conventional therapies – drugs and surgery – alone. An integrative approach, combining conventional and alternative therapies adapted to each patient, is aimed at promoting the healing of tissue and the elimination of pain rather than simply masking the problem with painkillers or, worse yet, surgery.

CHAPTER SIX

Conventional Approaches to Pain Treatment

Conventional medical treatment is very effective and should not be left aside in our eagerness to adopt alternative therapies. The combination of physical therapy and medications that I explain in this chapter provides our patients with prompt relief.

There is no single standard conventional medical treatment for arthritis, injuries and pain. Instead, there are many treatment options and modalities depending on the person and the type of problem. Different conditions, both acute and chronic, may involve slight or severe inflammation, very mild or advanced osteoarthritis, a clear history of recent injury or no injury at all. The pain felt by sufferers may be mild and in a small area, or intense and covering the whole arm or leg. This brings us to the following conclusions:

1. **Treatment must be adapted to the patient and not the patient to the treatment.** Rather than two or three structured treatment options for all cases, a wide variety of treatment options should be offered, coordinated, adapted and tried in each case. Both doctors and patients must understand this and keep an open mind when facing these challenges.

2. **Treatment should be provided not by one person but by a team.** This team should include a primary care doctor (who could be an internist, family or general practitioner, or chiropractor), and a group of other professionals. These could include a physical therapist, nutritionist, orthopedic doctor, chiropractor, rheumatologist, neurologist, and massage therapist, who may or may not be consulted according to the patient's needs. Other possible members of the team, depending on the patient's condition, could be an acupuncturist, reflexologist, podiatrist and the manager of the health food store. Both patients and physicians should have an open mind about calling on other professionals within both conventional and alternative medicine.

3. **The primary care doctor is not the sole provider of medical care to the patient.** Rather, he or she serves as the team coordinator. He or she will evaluate the patient and decide which of the above-listed consultants will be called in. He or she will explain the diagnosis and provide counseling to the patient, choose medications, arrange for appointments and follow-ups, and coordinate the care with the other professionals. He or she will be the captain of the ship, exercising command and control but understanding that treatment will not succeed without the efforts and goodwill of crew members.

4. **The use of medications, vitamins and supplements should never be liberal.** Excessive use of anti-inflammatories should be avoided, and the use of painkillers, although sometimes needed, should be controlled strictly. Vitamins and supplements should be limited to certain reliable brands. Careless use may provide no improvement and might even be harmful due to adverse reactions (see Chapter 9 for guidance).

5. **Patients and doctors alike need to increase their awareness of the alternative medicine providers in their area.** Integrative centers that combine conventional and alternative medicine already exist in many cities of the United

States. If integrative centers are not available, it is necessary to become acquainted with alternative medicine practitioners in the area. These practitioners need to be acknowledged, recognized, met with (in person), and even invited to be a part of an extramural team so that better choices are offered to the suffering patients. These practitioners are not competitors to the doctors, since they cannot treat the hundreds of conditions that only physicians can treat. These practitioners are, instead, doctors' helpers, assisting the physicians to achieve the main goal – to heal the patient.

The Jupiter Institute Pain Program of the *Jupiter Institute of the Healing Arts* (www.jupiterinstitute.com) was created with the idea of providing relief and of healing the condition in cases of pain, arthritis and injuries. It is an idea that works, although not every time. We invite physicians to follow our model, or the many other models like ours across the country, and to broaden the scope of their treatment options by counseling their patients about alternative medicine.

Patients need to understand that being pain-free requires personal effort and commitment. Healing will not come from a pill bottle or a surgeon's knife. Patients need to accept the fact that while pills provide relief, they are also hiding the problem. Although patients may feel better while taking the pills, their condition will be worsening if left untreated at its cause. Patients need to remember: **Pain is a message you should not ignore!**

CONVENTIONAL MEDICAL TREATMENT

Conventional medical treatment for arthritis, pain, and injury consists of a combination of the following:

1. Physical therapy
2. Medications
3. Exercise
4. Cortisone shots
5. Surgery

Physical Therapy

Physical therapy, also known as physical medicine and rehabilitation, is the most widely used treatment for arthritis, injuries and certain pains. It focuses on the reduction of inflammation and the recovery of function and attempts to suppress symptoms though physiologic healing. This patient-oriented emphasis on function rather than symptom suppression makes physical therapy the best treatment for all kinds of neuromuscular and skeletal disorders.

The role of physical therapy in treating pain, arthritis, and injures has expanded significantly over the last several years. Physical therapists work more closely with physicians and chiropractors, and improved communication has enhanced both treatment effectiveness and pain relief. Physical therapists have learned that early and effective application of pain-relieving modalities combined with patient education reduces many problems associated with pain, enabling individuals to resume their lifestyle much sooner.

Physical therapists are a mandatory addition to any therapy team as their knowledge and effectiveness makes them a vital component in any treatment plan.

Some of the physical therapy modalities include:

- **Heat therapy.** This can be applied using moist heat packs, paraffin baths, hot packs, heat lamps and hydrotherapy.

- **Ultrasound.** Ultrasound treatment can be given alone or using phonophoresis, which includes the addition of a steroid lotion that is forced into the tissues to increase treatment effectiveness. This technique uses an ultrasound device with a hand applicator.

- **Short wave and microwave diathermy** to provide deep heating of tissues.

- **Cold therapy (cryotherapy).** In this technique, cold packs are applied superficially to reduce blood flow, lessen muscle tone and decrease swelling. Treatment is rendered using ice, chemical packs or refrigerated units.

- **Transcutaneous Electrical Nerve Stimulator (TENS).** This is a small, cigarette-pack-sized device easily concealed in the pocket or under the belt and connected with wires and patches to the problem area. It provides pain relief but does not cure or heal.

- **Iontophoresis.** This therapy introduces substances through the skin and into deeper tissues using electrical paths.

- **Vibration.** This therapy is used to relax muscles in painful disorders.

- **Traction.** Traction is indicated for injuries of the cervical and lumbar spine. It can be accomplished through manual traction, mechanical traction or gravity traction. It is contraindicated in organic lesions of the spine: X-rays should be taken to eliminate these causes before starting treatment.

- **Compression.** The following are types of compression: ace wrapping, garments and gradient pumps.

- **Massage.** Massage stimulates nerve receptors producing muscular relaxation; it also improves blood flow to the muscle and stretches adhesions. Massage relieves pain, decreases swelling, and reduces muscle spasms.

- **Electrical stimulation.** Electrical stimulation speeds recovery in injured muscles. It also decreases spasm and pain.

- **Education.** The encounter between patient and therapist is unique. The patient has the special opportunity of being counseled on numerous aspects related to healing including exercise, avoidance of improper sports and incorrect posture, prevention of injuries, medications, and possible needs for consultations. Each one of these brief therapy sessions is a golden opportunity for the patient to receive some of the vast knowledge and expertise of the therapist.

- **Therapeutic exercise.** These are exercises taught by the therapist that the patient must perform at the therapy center or at home. They correct impairment and improve musculoskeletal function.

- **Aquatic therapy.** Pool therapy can be extremely beneficial, allowing exercise and improved relaxation.

Physical therapy is perhaps the most important of all patient treatments for neck and back pain, arthritis and injuries. By utilizing combinations of the above treatment modalities, therapists help to improve function, decrease stiffness, relieve pain and facilitate healing in the problem area. A course of physical therapy typically lasts only a few weeks, although long-term therapy may sometimes be recommended. Some excellent books are listed on our website (www.jupiterinstitute.com) for those who want to learn more.

Medications

Just as there is a variety of symptoms among people with arthritis, injury, and pain, there is a broad variety of medications to help control the symptoms. None of these medications heal; they merely decrease or eliminate the symptoms and provide temporary relief. However, anti-inflammatory medications, by slowing the process of inflammation, may occasionally prevent further damage caused by inflammation in the problem area.

In many circumstances, medications enhance the effect of physical therapy and increase the effectiveness of the treatment. The combination of Tylenol and an anti-inflammatory medication decreases the stiffness, swelling and pain caused by osteoarthritis, allowing millions of individuals to be able to have days of normal activity. Without these medications, these people would be prisoners of their daily stiffness, pain and disability. As much as these medications have been criticized, the benefits they provide are tremendous.

Although there are numerous arthritis and pain medications with exotic-sounding names, those most commonly used fall into one of these categories:

- Acetaminophen
- Non-steroidal anti-inflammatory drugs (NSAIDs)
- Corticosteroids
- Narcotic pain killers
- Topical pain relievers
- Muscle relaxants

ACETAMINOPHEN

You are probably familiar with acetaminophen. It is sold over the counter with brand names such as Tylenol, Datril, Panadol, etc. Many pharmacies have their own brand of acetaminophen.

Acetaminophen is a painkiller but is not anti-inflammatory, so it decreases pain but does not decrease inflammation. However, it is very effective for osteoarthritis pain, and among the safest drugs a patient with arthritis and pain can take. Considering the millions of doses consumed every year, it causes remarkably few side effects.

Acetaminophen does not act on the inflammation process of the joint and does not interact with the eicosanoids as the anti- inflammatory medications do. It works in the nervous system, decreasing the sensation of pain. Not messing with the eicosanoid system has both positives and negatives. The positives are that it does not interfere with the stomach eicosanoids, avoiding all the stomach problems that anti-inflammatories cause. The negatives are that it improves neither the eicosanoid imbalance nor the inflammation process at the problem areas.

Although not always effective, acetaminophen offers certain advantages:

- It is less expensive than a prescription medication.
- It is easily obtainable over the counter, found in grocery stores and gas stations around the world.
- It is gentle on the gastrointestinal tract and much less likely to cause a stomach to bleed or ulcer than some other medications.
- It will not raise blood pressure even after years of use.
- It is less likely to cause diseases of liver or kidney after many years.
- It is less likely to interact with other medications.

Despite its admirable safety record, acetaminophen can cause serious illness and liver damage and even death in large doses. Regular users need to know that they face an increased risk of liver and kidney damage. The risk of organ damage increases if the person consumes alcohol. Problems with acetaminophen almost always result from doses higher than the recommended 4,000 mg a day. It is critical to note that even moderate doses can be dangerous for older people and those with a liver disease. Most importantly, this medication (or any of the others) should not be used as a long-term strategy for managing pain. A full treatment program like the one outlined in this book is essential for the eradication of both pain, arthritis, and injury.

NON-STEROIDAL ANTI-INFLAMMATORY DRUGS (NSAIDs)

NSAIDs have become the most popular choice for physicians and patients when dealing with arthritis and pain. These first-line medications carry pain-killing properties, but they also slow down the production of the bad eicosanoids described earlier, which decreases the inflammation response. NSAIDs are effective for arthritic and injured patients and for all who suffer from pain. They come in over-the-counter products, prescription medications and even in injectable form. Intravenous NSAIDs are frequently given in the emergency department for numerous painful conditions.

NSAIDs have two names, one being the generic or pharmacological name and the other the brand name given by the pharmaceutical manufacturing company. The following are the most common NSAIDs being used, which are divided into three groups.

1. **Salicylates**
   Aspirin
   Sodium Salicylates (Salsalate, Trilisate)

2. **Non-selective COX inhibitors**
   Acetic acid derivatives
       Sulindac (Clinoril)
       Diclofenac Sodium (Voltaren)
       Diclofenac Potassium (Cataflam)
   Tolmetin (Tolectin)
   Indomethacin (Indocin)
   Propionic acid derivatives
       Ibuprofen (Motrin, Advil)
       Ketoprofen (Orudis, Oruvail)
       Fenoprofen (Nalfon)
       Oxaprozin (Daypro)
       Naproxen (Naprosyn, Aleve, Anaprox)
       Flurbiprofen (Ansaid)
   Oxicam derivatives
       Piroxicam (Feldene)
       Meloxicam (Mobic)
   Others
       Etodolac (Lodine)
       Ketorolac (Toradol)
       Nabumetone (Relafen)
       Meclofenamate (Ponstel)
       Diflunisal (Dolobid)

3. **Selective COX Inhibitors**
   Celecoxib (Celebrex) Rofecoxib (Vioxx)
   Valdecoxib (Bextra)

The anti-inflammatory action of the NSAIDs occurs at the level of the eicosanoids, also known as prostaglandins. We describe the whole inflammatory process in the chapter on inflammation. Inflammation, whether located in cartilage, ligament, tendons or muscle is a complex process of cell injury. "Good" eicosanoids are trying to decrease inflammation and heal the tissue while "bad" eicosanoids push for more inflammation and further tissue damage. In this process, arachidonic acid, which is a byproduct of omega fatty acids, interacts with the enzyme Cyclo-Oxygenase (COX) to produce eicosanoids.

There are two types of COX enzymes, COX-1 and COX-2. If the arachidonic acid interacts with COX-1, then good eicosanoids, which decrease inflammation and promote harmony in the local healing process, are produced. However, if the arachidonic acid reacts with COX-2, then bad pro-inflammatory eicosanoids are produced, intensifying and prolonging the inflammatory process.

Aspirin and all other NSAIDs non-selectively block both COX-1 and COX-2, reducing the total amount of all eicosanoids and blocking the inflammatory process. This decreases the swelling and pain, lowers the local temperature and lessens stiffness. It is important to note that NSAIDs decrease the *entire* inflammatory process, including the repair process. NSAIDs also decrease eicosanoid production in other areas. A lack of eicosanoids in the stomach, for example, causes a reduction in the secretions of the stomach's protective lining, making it susceptible to its own acidic juices. This is why NSAIDs can potentially cause stomach irritation, gastritis, ulcers, heartburn and even stomach bleeding. The use of NSAIDs is also linked to kidney damage.

The last group, selective COX inhibitors, work by selectively decreasing the action of the enzyme COX-2, therefore blocking the production of the bad pro-inflammatory eicosanoids and decreasing the swelling. This action results in the reduction of inflammation and pain.

COX-1 enzymes produce the protective mucus that coats the stomach and intestines. Regular NSAIDs have an adverse effect on both COX-1 and COX-2 enzymes, thereby decreasing this mucus secretion and thus promoting gastrointestinal irritation. However, COX-2 inhibitors do not affect gastrointestinal COX-1 enzymes, so the protective mucus is not harmed. That is how Celebrex, Vioxx and Bextra (the new COX-2 inhibitors) provide anti-inflammation without hurting the stomach. So, why was Vioxx removed from the market? Because it was hurting the COX enzymes that provide anti-inflammatory protection in the coronary arteries and in the heart, thus breaking the balance between eicosanoids and promoting coronary artery and heart disease. Celebrex and Bextra can cause coronary disease and heart attacks in the same way.

Advantages of COX-2 inhibitors. Cox-2 inhibitors are no more effective against pain and inflammation than standard NSAIDs. Their advantage lies in the lessening of gastrointestinal side effects, including irritation. They can also cause kidney damage like the other NSAIDs. However, COX-2 inhibitors are much more expensive than other NSAIDs.

Mobic and Relafen offer the advantage of providing mild COX-2 suppression, thus causing less gastrointestinal irritation in those who use them.

Side effects. Most side effects from NSAIDs are due to their inhibition of the "good" eicosanoids throughout the body. (See the description of "good" and "bad" eicosanoids in Chapter 3.) NSAIDs may disrupt the eicosanoids of the immune system, causing severe allergic reaction, in addition to high blood pressure, stomach irritation and bleeding. They can even trigger nausea, cramps, diarrhea, constipation, drowsiness, nervousness, asthma, dizziness, heart disease and kidney disorders. The longer the patient takes NSAIDs and the higher the dose, the more likely the side effects.

NSAIDs cause over 100,000 hospitalizations and lead to 16,000 deaths every year in America. If you want to learn more about the medications we recommend, we post the titles of several other books on our website (www.jupiterinstitute.com). Additional information about these medications may also be found in local libraries, bookstores, and the internet.

Two more disadvantages. There is growing evidence that NSAIDs may inhibit the synthesis of cartilage proteins, a vital part of the joint structure. This means that the same pill a person takes to relieve the symptoms of arthritis may cause further damage to an already arthritic joint.

The second disadvantage is the "wasting" effect. By decreasing and eliminating the symptoms of arthritis (pain, swelling and stiffness),

NSAIDs provide a false sense of improvement. Patients may then make two mistakes: they will not take care of a bad joint, and will continue performing activities that damage it, aggravating the injury even more. Considering this, NSAID use may actually worsen the osteoarthritis and injured area in the long run.

Advantages of NSAIDs: NSAIDs provide fast relief of pain, stiffness, swelling and disability. As a result, they are a good choice when treating numerous musculoskeletal disorders. Whether alone or combined with Tylenol, NSAIDs offer a handy and practical relief to headaches, pain and inflammation, improving the quality of life.

There are ways to prevent or minimize the adverse reaction caused by NSAIDs:

- Take them with food.
- Take them with a full 6 oz. glass of water.
- Do not lie down for at least 30 minutes.
- Do not take an excessive dose.
- At the first sign of stomach disturbance, take over-the-counter Pepcid or Maalox.
- Call your doctor as soon as possible if you feel any abnormal symptoms.
- Do not mix them with alcohol.
- Avoid taking them for a prolonged time periods.
- If you feel the need to take NSAIDs for longer periods, inform your doctor.

Using Aleve, Motrin IB, Advil or Ibuprofen is a very good idea on many occasions since it brings alleviation of symptoms without having to call a doctor or asking for assistance. But be extremely cautious with the amounts you take and the length of time you take them. Adverse reactions are like a tiger stalking you in the dark; any step can be a fatal one.

Corticosteroids

Corticosteroids, also known as steroids, include Prednisone, Medrol and the Steroid-Packs. They also come in injectable form and may be injected locally ("cortisone shots") or given intravenously. Steroids have a strong anti-inflammatory effect, which is much needed for many injuries, and for intense inflammation and pain conditions. They work very well. The main goal in using steroids is to stop the damaging effect of inflammation and the distress of severe pain. In these two areas, they do an excellent job. However, unless particular conditions require otherwise, steroids are short-course medications, used mainly to avoid an attack, crisis or sudden injury. They should be administered only by a physician.

Narcotic Pain Killers

Painkillers are by definition all those medications that decrease pain. We have already described the minor painkillers such as acetaminophen, aspirin, steroids and NSAIDs. We will now describe the major painkillers, also known as narcotics. Narcotics provide fast and effective pain relief, which is at times a very important issue when taking care of arthritis and injuries. They have an important role in the overall management of the suffering individual as they eliminate symptoms, allowing the person to resume a normal life and be able to sleep.

Some of the most common narcotics, alone or in a combination, are:

- Codeine (Tylenol #3, Tylenol #4)
- Fentanyl (Duragesic)
- Hydrocodone (Vicodin, Lorcet, Lortab, Vicoprofen, Annexa)
- Hydromorphone (Dilaudid)
- Levorphanol
- Meperidine (Demerol)
- Methadone (Dolophine)
- Morphine (MSIR, MS Contin, Kadian)

- Oxycodone (Roxicodone, OxyContin OxyIR, Percocet, Roxicet, Tylox)
- Oxymorphone (Numorphan)
- Propoxyphene (Darvon, Darvocet)

The disadvantage of narcotic painkillers is that they mask symptoms, fooling a person into thinking that the problem is actually healing when it may be getting worse. In addition, they have an enormous number of side effects, including addiction, sedation, constipation and respiratory depression. The list of the adverse reactions and drug interactions is very long and will not be presented here, but it is the responsibility of both the doctor and the patient to be aware of it. Doctors should instruct patients better about the side effects, but patients should not shield themselves behind the excuse of ignorance by saying, "My doctor never told me." Books on side effects of medications are found in most bookstores and libraries, and it is the responsibility of the patient to consult these information sources.

Nevertheless, as much as their use may be criticized, narcotics are often needed and recommended when treating severe pain. When used properly, they do provide relief and they do assist in the healing process. The type of narcotic, its dosage, and the length of treatment depend on the individual.

Topical Pain Relievers

These provide only local pain relief. They provide no healing. Some individuals apply them liberally to their problem areas and obtain a reduction in inflammation, pain and stiffness. This does not mean they provide any healing benefit to the injured tissues.

Muscle Relaxants

These medications are often used to treat muscle spasm associated with the injury of muscles, bones and joints. Other than in cases of severe spasm, they provide no benefit and generally should be avoided.

Exercise

Exercise helps keep the joints healthy while assisting in the healing process of joints, ligaments and muscles. However, certain exercises may actually be harmful to a joint or part of the body affected by arthritis, inflammation, injury or pain. Going for a five-mile walk with a sore knee or going to the gym to lift weights with an aching shoulder are common but unwise mistakes that need to be avoided. Improper exercise may amplify the damage and on occasion make it irreversible.

Physical therapists and chiropractors are the ideal professionals to consult about exercise. They can help you learn the exercises that may help in the healing process and those that should be avoided. (Note that physicians and orthopedic doctors are generally too busy to teach exercise to their patients.) You can find additional information about exercise in numerous books at the library and bookstores. We keep an updated list of recommended exercise books on our website (www.jupiterinstitute.com).

Surgery

On occasion, if all treatments fail, surgery is the only choice. The treating physician will then be in charge of recommending an appointment with an orthopedic doctor. Surgical procedures have clearly come a long way. The greatest surgical advances in the treatment of arthritis are joint replacement and arthroscopic surgery. Numerous joints can now be treated or replaced with new, refined surgical procedures. Orthopedic surgery is an excellent profession that provides relief to an enormous amount of patients. When appropriate, orthopedic surgery can be highly successful in providing relief.

Our Institute's Approach

We use medications as part of our treatment program, combining acetaminophen, anti-inflammatories and pain killers since they provide quick and effective relief. On occasion, we use corticosteroids as well. They are all part of our medical treatment, but we don't prescribe all or any of them to every person, we do not use them every time, and we do not give them in large doses. We use these medications because they provide unique relief and immediate comfort to the suffering patient, giving us time to coordinate the plan of treatment. Using medication with physical therapy also provides a prompt reduction of pain, giving the patient more time to think and make plans (you cannot think well when you are in pain). We then proceed to discuss the treatment plan with the patient, which includes the integration of chiropractic care, acupuncture, exercise and nutritional treatments.

CHAPTER SEVEN

A Nutrition Plan for Prevention and Treatment

 Diet has a major impact on arthritis, pain and inflammation, both as a cause and aggravator of these ailments, and as a course of prevention and treatment. A nutritionally balanced approach to food such as that offered by the Jupiter Institute Omega Diet may improve how a person feels and will likely also help to control the inflammatory process, often with unexpected side benefits to overall well-being.

An 81-year-old man named Tyson provides a good example of the overall positive impact afforded by our nutrition program. He was just days away from being placed in a nursing home by his three adult children when a neighbor told him about our program.

Accompanied by his children, Tyson came to see us and sat quietly as the two sons and daughter did most of the talking. They described how their father had severe arthritis and constipation. Most disturbing of all, his recent intellectual decline seemed to be a sign of senile dementia.

It took me quite a bit of persuasion to convince the four of them that our anti-inflammatory diet was the key to his recovery. When they were all finally in agreement, I drew up a list of aggravating foods and asked them to remove everything on the list from Tyson's kitchen and home. With our anti-inflammatory diet in place, I put him on nutritional supplements that included antioxidants and salmon gel caps. He also began daily sessions with our acupuncturist.

After just three weeks on our program, it was as if Tyson emerged from a mental fog and began to embrace an active life once again. The cloud of depression began to lift, his mind became sharper, the constipation disappeared, and he no longer had complaints about arthritis pain. He started reading the daily newspaper and went back to fishing. His laughter and sense of humor returned, and Tyson truly felt as if he had a new lease on life. None of his family members spoke ever again about the need for a nursing home.

In this chapter, you will learn about the composition and history of the diet that helped Tyson and many others recover. Understanding why and how this diet provides a healing and anti-inflammatory effect in the human body is an important step in appreciating the value of our program.

ONE OF THE BEST MEDICINES FOR TREATING THE INFLAMMATION OF ARTHRITIS AND INJURIES CAN BE FOUND NOT IN THE DRUGSTORE, BUT IN THE GROCERY STORE: THE PROPER FOOD

Many authorities agree that what we choose to put into our bodies can either strengthen or weaken us, making us more or less healthy while increasing or decreasing the symptoms of disease. Nutrition is known to affect the inflammation process. One of the best medicines for treating the inflammation of arthritis and injuries can be found, not in the drugstore but in the grocery store: the proper food.

Following dietary guidelines to improve arthritis, inflammation and pain has multiple advantages. Benefits include an improvement in the immune system's ability to fight infections and cancer, and improvements in both the cardiovascular system and glucose metabolism, decreasing the risks of heart attacks, diabetes and stroke.

The purpose of this diet is not to lose weight (although weight loss may come as a welcome secondary effect). Rather, it is a program designed to teach you about friendly and unfriendly foods that may trigger or relieve inflammation and pain.

Our dietary program consists of two parts:

1. Avoidance, which teaches you how to eliminate inflammation-causing foods, including foods with omega-6s, *and*
2. The Jupiter Institute Omega Diet, which tells you what foods help you reduce free radicals, and what foods help you increase your intake of antioxidants and omega-3s.

THE AVOIDANCE PLAN

Certain foods have a direct and toxic effect in inflammation and pain. Some of these foods provoke an allergic reaction while others act as toxic biochemical aggressors. There is evidence that particles of the foodstuffs listed below can cross the intestinal membrane, enter the blood stream, form immune complexes and then cause immuno-allergic injury in the tissues. By removing offending foods from the diet, people with painful conditions can avoid this adverse consequence and experience significant improvement in their symptoms.

Foods that cause arthritis, inflammation and pain:

- Chocolate
- Corn
- Dairy products
- Egg yolks
- Green and wax beans
- Milk
- Nightshade vegetables (eggplant, potatoes, green and red pepper, paprika and tomatoes)
- Nuts (mainly peanuts and sunflower seeds)
- Processed fruit juice
- Red meat
- Sugar
- Wheat and wheat flour
- Yeast and foods made with yeast

Our recommendation to avoid the above foods is based on numerous observations and reports of suffering people who removed these foods from their diet and found that their symptoms decreased while their quality of life improved. Wheat is a well-known trigger of arthritic conditions by provoking an allergic reaction to gluten. Gluten triggers an immuno-allergic type of response that can lead to inflammation and swelling.

Milk has been found to cause a variety of allergic reactions that cause inflammation and worsen arthritis.

The nightshade vegetables are strongly and consistently linked to arthritis. They contain chemicals that not only promote inflammation but also increase pain and interfere with the repair of damaged joints. Not many people get these immuno-allergic reactions, but those who do and suffer from pain and arthritis should stay away from nightshade vegetables.

In the same way, not every person is affected by immunotoxins such as wheat, milk, chocolate and sugar, but we recommend that those who suffer from pain, arthritis and other inflammation disorders stay away from these foods. Several weeks, perhaps a month later, a person can resume eating one or two of these products to see if the symptoms reappear. If they do not, they may be consumed infrequently and in small amounts.

Arthritis sufferers commonly have a high level of acidity, which is a fertile ground for inflammatory conditions. Acidity can be decreased by reducing the intake of acid-forming foods – such as these below – and switching to the Jupiter Institute Omega Diet.

Acid-forming foods

- Alcohol
- Beef
- Candy bars
- Cocoa
- Coffee
- Corn products (all)
- Flour products (all)
- Fried foods (all)
- Margarine
- Packaged snacks, chips
- Peanut butter
- Peanuts
- Pecans
- Sugar
- Sugary drinks & soft drinks
- Sweets
- Vinegar

THE JUPITER INSTITUTE OMEGA DIET

The Jupiter Institute Omega Diet is a program designed to improve health and decrease the rate of diseases, particularly those certain to affect people in the occidental world, such as arteriosclerosis, coronary heart disease, arthritis, vascular disease, and inflammatory diseases. The diet has a positive impact in the relief of osteoarthritis, inflammation and many other painful conditions.

The Jupiter Institute Omega Diet is based on the Mediterranean Diet – perhaps the healthiest traditional diet on the planet – with a few important differences. One difference, of course, is that people following this program know why they are eating what they are, unlike the people in the Mediterranean region who eat what they eat simply because of where they live! Another difference is that I have taken the 10 most important points of the Mediterranean Diet and explained, magnified and encouraged them. These 10 points have significant impacts on health, wellbeing and disease prevention.

The Jupiter Institute Omega Diet adds certain foods that increase the anti-inflammatory effects of the Mediterranean Diet while limiting or removing pro-inflammatory foods. I also recommend nutritional supplements and vitamins to enhance the healing effect of the Mediterranean Diet, decrease inflammation and arthritis, and promote repair and pain relief.

This combination of a healthy diet, plus nutritional addition, plus avoidance, provides a strong anti-inflammatory and pro-repair effect that assists in the management of injuries, arthritis, pain and inflammatory conditions.

Lastly, I have made our diet practical and easy to follow without the complications of puzzling cuisine and the confusion of strange names.

However, before you decide to follow this diet you must know why it will help you. Therefore, it is essential that you understand the heart of the Mediterranean Diet.

THE MEDITERRANEAN DIET

In the 1960s, a study called The Seven Country Study analyzed the diets and mortality of over 12,000 men in seven countries: The United States, Finland, Japan, Italy, Greece, Yugoslavia and The Netherlands. This study was long and complicated, and analyzed the causes of diseases and mortality in various age groups in these countries. The study showed that the healthiest participants lived in Japan and Greece. However, when comparing these two countries in greater detail, the Greeks were found to have a much lower rate of heart disease and greater longevity.

After analyzing the study and reviewing the Greek lifestyle, it was concluded that in defiance of conventional wisdom the Greeks who participated in the study achieved their low levels of heart disease risk despite endemic poverty, a poor healthcare system, and the consumption of a diet with the highest percentage of fat.

The United States, with its great healthcare system, wealth, excellent supermarkets and wide availability of processed food, take-out restaurants, fast food and its surplus of eating choices, did very poorly in this study. It also showed much lower longevity and an excessive rate of heart attacks, strokes and inflammatory conditions to begin with. The contrast with the findings in Greece was dramatic.

The amazing results of the clinical studies of the Greek population led to a further investigation that extended to other countries of the Mediterranean region. For over 40 years, public health officials have been studying the diets of the Mediterranean. The people in Greece have been found to derive the greatest benefits from this type of diet, followed by southern Italy, Spain and France.

The Mediterranean area is bordered by three continents – Europe, Africa and Asia – and embraces more than a dozen countries. Regions that influence the Mediterranean Diet include Portugal, Southern Spain, Southern France, Southern Italy, Greece, Southern Turkey, Lebanon, Western Syria, Western Israel, Northern Egypt and the northern regions of Morocco, Libya and Algeria.

The important aspects of the Mediterranean Diet are:

- High intakes of fish, olives, olive oil, grains, fresh vegetables, beans, garlic, fresh herbs and fresh fruits.
- Poultry in moderation and red meat occasionally.

- Abundance of food from plant sources (fruits, vegetables, beans, grains and rice).
- Minimally processed, seasonally fresh and locally grown foods.
- A high consumption of good fat (olive oil, olives, fish and nuts being the principal sources of fat).
- Low consumption of low-fat cheeses and yogurts (which are used mainly as condiments).
- Fish, poultry and eggs as the main protein.
- Nuts and fresh fruits are a typical daily dessert.
- Moderate consumption of wine, especially red wine.
- Olives and nuts for appetizers and snacks.

The traditional Mediterranean Diet is affected by regions and seasons. While each Mediterranean country has its customs, they all rely on locally or regionally grown produce, consumed shortly after harvest. Every season provides fresh new vegetables that are often eaten within a few miles of where they were picked.

Outdoor markets offer fresh fruits and vegetables and plenty of locally produced olive oil. The consumption of all these products in their freshest state is one of the important features of the local meals.

For more detail on the Mediterranean Diet, see the recommended books listed on our website (www.jupiterinstitute.com).

Key Benefits

Hundreds of articles have been published in medical and scientific journals about clinical research on the Mediterranean Diet. Most of this research shows that adherence to the Mediterranean Diet improves health and longevity, prevents heart and vascular disease, improves arthritis, heals injuries, relieves pain and even prevents cancer. It also has a powerful anti-inflammatory effect, which has a positive impact on the treatment of arthritis and inflammatory conditions of muscles, tendons and ligaments.

Despite a higher fat intake, people in Mediterranean countries show better overall health and longer life expectancy. They suffer less from arthritis and pain, and their injuries even heal better and with less distress. The diet has a beneficial effect on fatigue and psychological disorders such as anxiety and depression.

The beneficial effect of the Mediterranean Diet on heart disease is dramatic. This diet prevents heart attacks, but if a person has already had one, this diet will prevent or delay the onset of a second heart attack. It can also lower blood pressure and prevent atherosclerosis.

Additionally, this diet has a dramatic effect on the joints. It prevents arthritis, and if a person is already suffering from arthritic conditions, it promotes healing and decreases inflammation of the affected joints. The same thing is true with injuries. Injuries, whether from a car accident, surgery or trauma, heal better and faster when following the Mediterranean Diet.

The same occurs for those suffering with fatigue, body aches, and psychological disorders such as mood swings, anxiety, depression, and even Alzheimer's disease. Those who are already affected by these conditions do better on this diet and experience a significant reduction of symptoms and an overall improvement in the quality of life.

Although the term "Mediterranean Diet" implies that all Mediterranean people eat the same foods, of course this is not so. The countries of the Mediterranean Sea have different diets, religions and cultures. Their diets differ in the amount of fat, protein, grains, types of meat and wine intake. However, extensive studies show that although the diet may vary from country to country, the overall benefit does not change much. Pasta is eaten in some Mediterranean countries, but not in others; sourdough bread or more cheese is eaten in some; lamb in some, not in others; goat in some, in others only fish and poultry.

The type and quantity of nuts and vegetables also varies, but these are just variations within the same type of diet. In total, the Mediterranean people who follow this way of eating do not eat vegetable oil or salad dressing, hamburgers or fried food, pizza, martinis, beer, chips, dips or excessive beef. Unlike people in North America and Northern Europe, they do not consume excessive quantities of saturated fat (from animal products), trans fatty acids (from hydrogenated oils in manufactured and processed food), omega-6 fatty acids (from dairy, corn, meat and bakery products) and processed carbohydrates. However, consumption of omega-3 foods (fish, nuts and vegetables) and omega-9 foods is high. Instead of having an unhealthy ratio of omega-6 to omega-3 of 20, 30 or even 40 to 1, as in the United States, the ratio is about 3 to 1, which is very good for general health and especially good for preventing cardiovascular disease, arthritis and even cancer.

The effect on the omega fatty acid balance is perhaps the most important factor of the Mediterranean Diet and the one that provides the greatest health benefit. High intake of omega-3 fatty acids from fish, vegetables and nuts, coupled with the consumption of powerful antioxidants from herbs, fruits, wine and vegetables places people in an omega-3/antioxidant state, which provides tremendous health benefits, unlike the omega-6/free-radical state of the American diet, which is toxic, extremely inflammatory and disease-causing.

The Cardiovascular Advantage

Over the last 15 years, many studies have focused on unveiling the metabolic pathways through which the Mediterranean Diet provides its benefits. Among their conclusions is that such a diet:

1. **Lowers overall cholesterol levels.**

2. **Raises levels of HDL** (high-density lipoprotein), which is the good cholesterol that provides cardiovascular protection.

3. **Lowers levels of LDL** (low-density lipoprotein), which is the bad cholesterol that causes heart and vascular disease.

4. **Reduces the oxidation of LDL,** making it less prone to harden the arteries (atherogenic). This means that even if the LDL is elevated, the Mediterranean Diet protects the coronary and vascular system against its bad effects. In a way, the Mediterranean Diet shields the body against the bad effect of LDL.

5. **Lowers the CRP (C-reactive protein),** which is a marker of the degree of inflammation in the vascular system. High CRP indicates active inflammation in the blood vessels and indeed throughout the body; it is currently used as a marker to indicate the progression of cardiovascular disease and atherosclerosis. CRP is considered a high risk factor for heart disease. Research shows that individuals affected by high levels of CRP are more affected by the devastating effects of atherosclerosis, which includes peripheral vascular disease (lack of circulation in the legs), heart attacks, strokes and many other conditions. Current cardiovascular preventive practices recommend lowering the levels of CRP. The Mediterranean Diet, as evidenced by publication in many journals and books, offers the beneficial effect of lowering C-reactive protein levels.

6. **Reduces the risk of atherosclerosis.** The Mediterranean Diet affects the eicosanoid system, increasing the presence and actions of good (anti-inflammatory) eicosanoids and reducing bad (pro-inflammatory) eicosanoids. The eicosanoids are like super-hormones that control tissue metabolism. As we have noted, good eicosanoids decrease inflammation, increase the healing and repair and prevent diseases. Bad eicosanoids damage tissue, cause inflammation and pain, and promote arthritis, aches, stiffness, atherosclerosis and many other major diseases, including immune diseases and metabolic disease. They worsen diabetes, elevate blood pressure and even promote obesity.

The Lyon Diet Heart Study

This study of the benefits of the Mediterranean Diet was published in 2001. It tested the effects of the Mediterranean Diet on the recurrence of coronary disease attacks after a first myocardial infarction (heart attack). A total of 605 patients was randomized in the study. Of them, 303 patients were given the diet recommended by the American Heart Association (also recommended by many medical doctors, cardiologists and dietetic associations in the United States), and 302 were instructed to follow the Mediterranean Diet that contained many grains, vegetables, olive oil, nuts, abundant fish and fruits and even moderate amounts of red wine with meals.

After 27 months of follow-up, this Lyon Diet Heart Study was ended early by the Ethics Committee because of the significant difference in coronary attacks between the two groups. The beneficial effect of the Mediterranean Diet on heart attacks was such that it was unfair for those following the American diet to continue the study; they were dying in excess. Despite the similar coronary risk factor profile, those on the Mediterranean Diet had approximately 60% lower incidence of recurrent coronary attacks, and the difference in hospitalization was just as impressive. While those following the Mediterranean Diet were enjoying life, the Americans were dying like flies.

The Lyon Diet Heart Study illustrates the importance of the dietary pattern in the prevention and treatment of heart disease. One of the conclusions of the study was that omega-3 and omega-9 fatty acids, which are in abundance in the Mediterranean Diet, exert a powerful heart-protection effect. This cardio-protective effect is due to their activities in preventing rhythm disturbance in the heart, their anti-inflammatory effect, their anti-clotting effect, their effect in lowering toxic products at the coronary artery wall, their effect of lowering bad eicosanoids and increasing good eicosanoids, and their ability to inhibit atherosclerosis.

The study concluded that the public health benefit of the Mediterranean Diet is enormous.

Effects on Inflammation and Pain

The Mediterranean Diet has a potent anti-inflammatory effect, the result of its omega-3 content. Arthritis and joint disease are less common in people following the Mediterranean Diet. When people who are affected by advanced osteoarthritis are placed on this diet, swelling decreases, and spinal stiffness and general healing improves. Painful conditions such as neck, back and joint pain improve significantly as well.

Injury sufferers (from car accidents, trauma, and surgery) heal better when following the Mediterranean Diet, thanks to its beneficial metabolic effect. Sports injuries heal faster too, which is why many trainers use it to treat injured athletes.

The anti-inflammatory effect of this diet also protects against coronary atherosclerosis and coronary obstruction, reducing the risk of sudden cardiac death. Other conditions including allergies, asthma, PMS, menstrual cramps, headaches, skin disorders, neuropathy, mood disorders and irritable bowels also get significant relief from the Mediterranean Diet.

MORE ABOUT KEY ELEMENTS OF THE MEDITERRANEAN DIET

Olive oil

For centuries, the nutritional and medicinal benefits of olive oil have been recognized by the people of the Mediterranean region. Recent research has confirmed what the Mediterranean people already knew – that olive oil prevents and heals many diseases, promotes health and increases longevity.

Olive oil is the principal source of fat in the Mediterranean Diet. Because of its chemical structure, olive oil is unrivaled in its value and, thus, the oil best suited for human consumption. It is also extremely well tolerated by the stomach and intestines, where it actually exerts a protective function. The excellent digestibility of olive oil promotes the overall absorption of nutrients, especially vitamins and minerals.

Olive oil helps sustain human metabolism at a sensible balance and provides the body with good vitamin E. Studies at university centers showed that olive oil decreases the oxidative state of the LDL, the bad cholesterol, making it less harmful to the vascular system. An even more important finding of these studies is that olive oil decreases the production of arachidonic acid, the father of all bad eicosanoids. The omega-6 foods that we mentioned in another section of this chapter produce arachidonic acid, which in turn generates the bad eicosanoids responsible for inflammation, disease and pain.

Olive oil reduces the formation of arachidonic acid by inhibiting a specific enzyme called delta-6-desaturase. This action makes olive oil a powerful anti-inflammatory agent that provides benefits at every level of the body. It is especially beneficial in many degenerative inflammatory processes including osteoarthritis, inflammatory arthritis, injuries, and other painful conditions.

Olive oil has been the most distinguished element of Mediterranean cooking for thousands of years. Although Spanish and Italian olive oil dominates international markets, Greek olive oils are excellent products as well. Extra virgin olive oil has a long shelf life and is best for salads and salad dressings. Other types of olive oil can be used for frying, but our recommendation is not to eat fried foods or foods cooked with a lot of olive oil. It is best to consume olive oil in its natural, uncooked state, straight from the bottle drizzled lightly on your food.

Red Wine

In studies involving many thousands of participants, red wine consumption has been shown to reduce the risk of death from coronary disease and cancer. Studies also show that red wine, but no other alcoholic beverage, decreases cardiovascular mortality. The habit of moderate consumption of wine has been found to increase longevity.

Concerns have been expressed by certain social and religious groups regarding the drinking of wine and a possible association with alcohol abuse, liver disease and dependency. Nevertheless, studies show that when consumed responsibly, red wine is beneficial for the cardiovascular system and an important component of a healthy lifestyle. The Diet recommends one or two servings of 2-4 ounces each during a meal.

North Europeans, who became upset with the news of the benefits of wine, performed clinical studies to test whether whiskey, beer and other alcoholic beverages were as beneficial for the cardiovascular system as red wine. These studies ended in profound defeat, showing that alcoholic beverages other than red wine actually increase cardiovascular disease. Only red wine has been shown to protect health and provide health benefits. (White wine was defeated as well.)

The beneficial effects of red wine occur through several pathways:

- Its antioxidant effect, which neutralizes free radicals and protects the HDL (the good cholesterol), preventing vascular and tissue damage.
- Its boosting of HDL levels (the higher the HDL, the lower the risks for heart attack).
- Its vasodilating effect (dilatation of small arteries).
- Its anti-clogging effect prevents the formation of blood clots that block the coronary arteries.
- Its relaxing effect decreases stress and psychological tension.
- The extraordinary amount of nutrients it contains, including flavonoids, antioxidants, and resveratrol, are anti-inflammatory, anti-clogging and anti-cancerous.
- The daily consumption of one or two glasses of red wine does not appear to have any harmful effect other than adding calories to the diet.

Numerous epidemiological studies, including the Copenhagen Health Study, the Nurses' Heart Study, the Framingham Study, and the American Cancer Society Study associate moderate red wine consumption with health and longevity.

Much can be said about the excellent combination of red wine and olive oil. However, for the sake of time and space, we will focus on the entire Mediterranean Diet.

Natural Antioxidants

One of the highlights of the Mediterranean Diet is its high content of natural antioxidants.

The health benefits of antioxidants are well known. They neutralize toxic free radicals, which are molecules that cause inflammation and damage in our tissues. Free radicals oxidize and neutralize the

HDL (the good cholesterol) and cause damage in joints and injured areas, worsening arthritis and pain. Antioxidants counteract these effects by blocking the free radicals. Therefore, they enhance healing and repair of injuries, decrease pain and improve both arthritis and coronary inflammation.

The sources of these nutrients in the Mediterranean Diet are:

- Plant food, fresh legumes and vegetables consumed uncooked.
- Red wine.
- Fresh herbs (basil, bay leaves, chives, cilantro, dill, fennel, garlic, marjoram, oregano, parsley, rosemary, sage, thyme, tarragon and others). You can get them at the supermarket or in pots at garden stores.
- Fresh raw fruits.

In addition to their protective effect on HDL and tissues, antioxidants also protect omega-3 fatty acids from being destroyed by free radicals.

The intake of antioxidants in their fresh, natural state is mandatory and essential for good health. Awareness of this issue is very important. Antioxidants can be ingested through the foods we mentioned above, but frequently this consumption is not sufficient and the use of vitamins and supplements is, therefore, recommended. This will be explained further when we get to the basic concepts of the Jupiter Institute Omega Diet. Supplements and vitamins are discussed in more detail in Chapter 9.

Fish And Fish Oil

Eicosapentaenoic acid (EPA) and docosahexaenoic acid (DHA) are the omega-3 fatty acids in fish that provide tremendous health benefits to joints, organs and to the cardiovascular system. However, qualities vary greatly depending on the species of fish, whether the fish was farm-raised or caught in the deep cold ocean, and whether it is eaten raw, cooked or canned. This is discussed in more detail later in this chapter.

The benefits of the diet consumed by Mediterranean people come largely from the abundance of alpha linoleic acid, phytochemicals, natural vitamins and minerals (not man-made vitamin pills), carotenoids, lycopene, glutathione, antioxidants, and many other natural nutrients. All of these provide enormous health advantages to the human body.

These beneficial effects are even more pronounced in an enhanced Mediterranean Diet plan, such as our Jupiter Institute Omega Diet. Larger amounts of these helpful biochemicals are available in a more standardized way, and with more regularity.

THE JUPITER INSTITUTE OMEGA DIET IN BRIEF

Foods That Are Best To Eat

Listed below are the food groups we recommend you eat. You will find omega-3 fatty acids in items 1, 2, 3, 5, 6, 10 and 11. You will find the antioxidants in items 7, 8A, 9, 10 and 11.

1. **Protein.** White protein is best, but yellow is acceptable. The best white protein is found in fish, egg whites, Egg Beaters, boxed egg whites, lean chicken, lean turkey (white meat), tofu, fat-free cottage cheese and fat-free dairy products (a whole egg a day is okay, too). Yellow proteins, such as low-fat cheese, are also acceptable.

   Remember that although you need protein every day you do not need a lot. Excess protein is not good, and neither is a protein-free diet. Brown rice combined with beans is a very good source of protein. We strongly recommend that you eat your protein with some vegetables and olive oil. Pork and pork products, as well as veal, are not recommended. Beef and lamb can be consumed once a week, which is enough. Cold cuts like salami, ham, pepperoni and bologna are not advisable. Cold cuts of chicken, turkey and pastrami can be consumed mainly for lunch, but only in minimal amounts.

2. **Fish.** Eat fish regularly! The best kinds are oily fish: anchovies, bluefish, cod, halibut, herring, mackerel, salmon, sardines, tuna, and trout.

   Raw fish is better than cooked, and cooked is better than canned. Canned fish in water mixed with additional olive oil is better than fish canned in oil.

   Fish caught in the deep ocean waters contain much more omega-3 fatty acids than farmed fish because deep ocean fish feed on algae, which is rich in omega-3. However, they are not always easy to get. Market conditions, distribution and price often make it more convenient and practical to obtain farm-raised fish. Although farm-raised fish are not a panacea, they are often subject to overcrowding, disease and other deleterious conditions. Make sure you inquire about the source of your fish whenever possible.

   The white, flaky, non-oily fish (such as grouper, snapper, mahi-mahi and cobia from Florida), are good sources of protein but contain no omega-3.

   King mackerel, kingfish and swordfish do contain omega-3, but I do not recommend them: first, they may be contaminated with mercury (see the sidebar later in this chapter); second, I feel sorry for the swordfish, which are often victims of trophy hunters.

   Variations in omega-3 fatty acids also occur in tuna. Tuna, when eaten raw and fresh, offers significant amounts of it, but canned tuna, which has been cooked at least twice in the process of packing, has much less.

3. **Olive oil and olives (green and black).** Only extra virgin oil is recommended. We do not recommend light olive oil. One or two tablespoons of regular extra virgin oil twice a day is the current recommendation – uncooked oil that goes straight from the bottle to the food. (Cooked oils are best to avoid as they do not have nearly the same health benefits as uncooked oils, and could be harmful. If you cook oil, make sure that it is fresh oil and that you are only cooking in it for a few minutes at most.) Olives, either green or black, are strongly recommended, as garnish for food, and as a snack.

    For variety, you can flavor your oil, combining it with lemon juice and salt, thyme and oregano, or with chopped fresh herbs. Alternatively, you can mix it with a little French mustard, ketchup and horseradish, barbecue sauce or fat-free mayonnaise, or mix it with a combination of dry herbs.

4   **Natural grains, beans and pulses.** Recommended grains are rice, brown rice, couscous, quinoa, and even bulgur, as well as "pseudograins" such as quinoa and millet, which are actually not grains but seeds from plants. Recommended pulses (legumes) and beans are lentils and dried beans (canned beans are OK as long as they are plain), green beans and string beans.

    Green peas and chickpeas are allowed – but only in small amounts and only on occasion. Intake should be limited because chickpeas and green peas have excessive carbohydrates and unwanted amounts of omega-6s. Although hummus is a typical Mediterranean dish, it is traditionally consumed in small quantities. You should eat it only on rare occasions and in small amounts. The reason is the preparation: in Mediterranean countries, hummus is prepared with a large amount of fresh olive oil while the tendency in the United States is to use processed oils and other preservatives. Hence, because of its high omega-6 content, it is not recommended. This recommendation does not apply as strictly to homemade hummus prepared with fresh olive oil; still, care should be taken not to over-consume it.

Corn is full of omega-6s and should be avoided.

Consume grains in their natural forms. Avoid processed products of the grains we mention here, such as rice cakes, rice crackers, refried beans, bean dips, processed lentil soups, processed pea soups, and so on.

5. **Nuts.** Walnuts are the nuts that we recommend the most, although macadamia nuts, pumpkin seeds, almonds and hazelnuts are also approved.

   Brazil nuts, cashews and pecans are not recommended. Peanuts are not nuts, and they are forbidden. Sesame seeds and sunflower seeds are seeds, not nuts, and are forbidden as well. All by-products of these "nuts" – peanut oil, peanut butter, sesame oil, tahini, safflower oil, and pecan products – are not allowed.

6. **Flaxseeds.** Flaxseeds, ground flaxseeds, flaxseed oil and flaxseed gel caps are strongly recommended and should be liberally consumed. Feel free to use them as often as you want and in the quantities you desire. They are an excellent source of omega-3.

7. **Red wine.** Red wine is the only alcohol allowed in the Jupiter Institute Omega Diet. It is approved in quantities of 2-4 ounces at a time and with a meal only. One time a week, at home, at dinnertime is a good way to begin.

   As with any alcoholic drink, one should be aware of the side effects and act responsibly. Consuming alcohol is not required for health. However, if you wish to drink wine, consume it always at dinnertime and in the stipulated quantities of 2-4 ounces. No driving is allowed after consumption. (Being aware of the adverse effects of using alcohol while on medication is the responsibility of the patient. You must consult your doctor.)

8. **Herbs.** Herbs contain minerals and antioxidants that are not found in any other food and are crucial to our metabolism. Fresh herbs also provide valuable vitamins.

   Here is a list of common herbs:
   - Basil
   - Bay leaves
   - Chives
   - Cilantro
   - Coriander
   - Dill
   - Garlic
   - Ginger
   - Marjoram
   - Mint
   - Oregano
   - Parsley
   - Rosemary
   - Thyme

   Fresh raw herbs have a much higher concentration of antioxidants; that is why we recommend them. You can find them in plastic containers or bags in the vegetable section of the supermarket. You can also buy them in pots at garden stores and plant them in your backyard. Try getting into the habit of using fresh herbs regularly in your salad. Adding fresh herbs and olive oil to your salad is a very healthy habit. When fresh herbs cannot be obtained, dried herbs are acceptable.

9. **Raw fruit.** Raw fruit is strongly recommended. A variety of seasonal fruit is best. Your local market is one source, but look for fruit that has been recently picked. Fruit that has been picked too many days in advance has lost much of its antioxidant and vitamin value. One of the best examples is the bananas found in local American markets, which have been picked green many

days and even weeks ahead. By the time they are consumed by the public, by now yellow and soft, their vitamin and antioxidant content is very low. Other examples are mangoes and oranges. They, too, have been harvested too many days before reaching the market. Even though they have been refrigerated, their vitamin and antioxidant content is low. Each market in each state is different. The reader needs to take into account the possible local production and the origin of each of the fruits they find. Again, local fruits in season and picked when ripe are best.

10. **Vegetables.** Fresh and raw is best. Vegetables can be steamed, but just lightly. The more a vegetable is cooked, the lower its vitamin and antioxidant content. A variety of vegetables and vegetables of different colors are strongly recommended. Frozen vegetables are okay, but their vitamin and antioxidant content is also very low. All fresh vegetables are a source of good (complex) carbohydrates, natural vitamins and antioxidants. Some have a high omega-3 content, which makes them desirable for those who follow our program. These omega-3 vegetables are:

- Alfalfa sprouts
- Arugula
- Bean sprouts
- Broccoli
- Cauliflower
- Collard greens
- Kale
- Lettuce
- Mustard greens
- Romaine
- Spinach
- Watercress

Corn and potatoes are not allowed.

11. **Recommended vitamins and supplements.** These are capsules and tablets including omega-3 fatty acids (fish oil, salmon oil, flaxseed oil), gamma-linoleic acid (GLA), antioxidants and vitamins. See Chapter 9 for guidance.

12. **Avoidance.** Whatever is not listed above should be avoided – especially omega-6 food including fried food, sugary baked goods, and processed food as discussed later in this chapter.

Additional recommendations for the Jupiter Institute Omega Diet

1. **Snacks.** Learn to snack on things you can have – walnuts, olives, fruits, or a bit of bread dipped in olive oil. Canned mushrooms, canned beans, canned heart of palms and canned asparagus are also acceptable.

   Snacks to avoid: if you do not see an item on my list, ask your doctor or chiropractor, or contact us by phone, mail or fax. Sugar, honey and alcohol other than wine are not allowed.

2. **Beware of marketing.** Foods you see in television commercials are bad for you. If you see someone on television in a white coat pushing a particular food, he or she is being paid to mislead you. Much of the food advertising in magazines is misleading and manipulative. Be careful!

3. **Go easy on:** Soy sauce and diet sodas – these are OK, but only rarely. Pasta is allowed one to three times a month, and no more. Two slices of bread a day is allowed. A little fruit spread (with no added sugar) for your toast and a little milk for your coffee are also allowed. One or two cups of coffee in the morning are OK, but not more than that.

4. **Do eat fat!** But it must be good fat, like that found in nuts, olive oil and avocado. Never eat fat-free meals and never touch deep-fried food!

5. **Restaurants are dangerous.** With some exceptions, restaurants are dangerous for your diet. Do not waste your time, your money or your health on such foods. Cruises are also not healthy because of the uncontrolled amounts of food that people have a tendency to consume. Do not go places where your dietary plan will be in danger.

6. **Read labels.** If the fat content of a food product you are buying is more than zero percent, then you can be sure it contains processed fat, which is bad for your body.

7. **Not recommended:** Salami, pepperoni, mozzarella cheese, hamburger, shakes, pizza, fried chicken, potato salad, coleslaw, supermarket salads, hot dogs, pâté, cheeses, luncheon meats, sour cream, milk, frozen dinners, chain-restaurant "Mexican" food, chili, bagels, cream cheese, donuts, muffins, pastries, cakes, ice cream, candy bars, peanuts, peanut butter, bakery products, butter, margarine, salad dressing, commercial sauces, liquor, beer, chips and dips, and any food from fast-food restaurants such as Wendy's, Taco Bell, McDonald's and Burger King.

8. **Manufactured and processed food.** If the food was made in a factory or a restaurant, it was not made with your health in mind.

9. **Cereal products.** Whole wheat bread (not recommended because of the gluten: use gluten-free breads if need be), oatmeal, breakfast cereal and granola are inventions to make you believe you are eating healthfully. I do not recommend them. They are not included in the Mediterranean Diet.

10. **Certain vegetable oils.** Corn oil, sunflower oil, safflower oil, cottonseed oil, peanut oil and sesame oil are not good for you. They are even worse when cooked or fried.

Mercury contamination in fish: cause for concern?

Unfortunately, many types of fish are contaminated with mercury. Mercury pollution in lakes, rivers and oceans ends up accumulating in the flesh of certain types of fish. Not all fish are contaminated. Within the same species, some are contaminated and some are not. Depending on their origin, salmon and tuna, for example, may be slightly or very contaminated, or not contaminated at all.

Excessive consumption of fish contaminated with mercury can lead to mercury poisoning.

Cooking does not remove the mercury from the fish because it is bound to the flesh. Hence, a piece of tuna will have the same amount of mercury whether you bake it, grill it or eat it as sushi.

In 2004, the FDA and the U.S. Environmental Protection Agency (EPA) issued an advisory recommending that women who are or might become pregnant, nursing mothers and young children should not eat shark, swordfish, king mackerel or tilefish because they contain high levels of mercury. In addition, people in these same groups should limit their consumption of fish and shellfish with lower mercury content to 12 oz. per week (two average meals).

More recently, however, a study from the National Institutes of Health suggested that the benefits for unborn babies of the omega-3 fatty acids contained in fish eaten by their mothers outweigh the risks to their development posed by the mercury content.

We cannot offer hard and fast guidelines about what types of fish to eat, and how much, in order to avoid the dangers of mercury contamination.

On the other hand, I think we can take courage from these recent findings of the NIH. Clearly, it would be wise to avoid eating the kinds of fish containing the highest levels of mercury. But in my view it is equally wise to eat regular, but not excessive, portions of other kinds, particularly those high in omega-3 fatty acids.

We encourage you to ask in the supermarket and consult your local authorities to learn more about this issue. You can also search on the internet, or call local agencies or poison control centers.

THE OMEGA-3/ANTIOXIDANT STATE

The Jupiter Institute Omega Diet combines three key elements:

1. The Mediterranean Diet.

2. Avoidance of foods with omega-6s and activators of omega-6.

3. Supplements of omega-3s and carefully chosen antioxidants (see Chapter 9).

This diet is designed to elevate you into the omega-3/antioxidant state that we emphasize for reduced pain and inflammation.

The foods we eat, the supplements we take, and our own lifestyle habits (exercise, sleep, etc.) can balance the metabolism (what we call the omega-3/antioxidant state) or cause imbalance (what we call the pro-inflammatory omega-6/free-radical state). Both of these metabolic conditions work through activating – favorably or unfavorably – the eicosanoid system that we described earlier. In the omega-3/antioxidant state all metabolic functions work in harmony, so inflammation, cellular damage and pain are decreased.

The omega-3/antioxidant state has these benefits:

- **In joints:** the symptoms of arthritis-like swelling, pain and stiffness decrease. Chronic discomfort in joints and muscles is reduced as inflammation in tendons and joints improves. Motion restrictions decrease and the need for medications diminish.

- **In pain situations:** headaches and migraines become less frequent and less intense. Neck pain, back pain, pain from injury, and arthritic pain are significantly alleviated.

- **In the vascular system:** coronary inflammation decreases while episodes of angina decrease and become less frequent. Blood pressure improves, and hypertension is better regulated.

- **In the lungs:** asthma improves – attacks become less frequent and less intense.

- **In the muscular system:** injuries from accidents and athletic injuries heal better and with less pain.

- **In diabetes:** glucose control improves. Need for diabetic medication, including insulin, decreases.

- **In high cholesterol situations:** levels of HDL – the good cholesterol – rise, and levels of LDL – the bad cholesterol – fall, providing a better risk ratio.

- **In psychological conditions:** irritability and anxiety decrease, while depression improves. People become calmer.

- **In the gastrointestinal system:** fewer and milder abdominal cramps from IBS (irritable bowel syndrome).

- **Other benefits:** thyroid function becomes more stable; neuralgias become less painful; acne and eczema improve, and symptoms of chronic fatigue lessen.

THE IMPORTANCE OF WHAT YOU DON'T EAT

When it comes to healthy eating, what people don't eat is just as important as what they do eat. Meat, in general, carries a lot of saturated fat and other substances that pose a threat to health. Some of these substances are known to generate cardiovascular diseases and cancer. Mediterranean people consume very little meat, if any, and avoid seed oils such as corn, sunflower, cottonseed and soybean oil. They also consume very little butter and milk and avoid the dense fatty acids of margarine, processed food, frozen meals and snacks.

Food such as cheese, pizza, cheeseburgers, a glass of milk, meat and potatoes, bagels with cream cheese, hot dogs, barbecued ribs, breakfast cereal, orange juice, mayonnaise, cookies, ice cream, and many other foods typical of the American diet, are not consumed by Mediterranean people. In general, they do not expose themselves to large steaks, pork products, large pasta dishes, shakes, luncheon meats, donuts, beer, chips, dips and salad dressings. They do not embrace the typical American breakfast, brunch buffets, waffles, pancakes and the great variety of breads and cereals commonly consumed in the United States. Therefore, they don't load themselves with saturated fat, fried food, processed foods that are high in refined carbohydrates, and trans fatty acids, which are loaded with toxic, pro-inflammatory omega-6s.

As compensation for a more simple and natural way of eating, Mediterraneans are rewarded with better health, fewer strokes and heart attacks, and less arthritis and cancer. They also live longer. However, Mediterraneans who depart from their traditional diet and adopt foods from other cultures – specifically Northern Europe and the U.S. – do not do well. The significant increase in omega-6 fatty acids causes these Mediterraneans to develop the same diseases (atherosclerosis, inflammation and vascular diseases) as the cultures who eat this way. When Mediterranean people – regardless of where they live – don't follow a Mediterranean Diet, their health suffers. So, if Mediterraneans eat like Americans, they die like Americans.

PROCESSED FOODS

Processed foods are made in a factory from once-natural and whole foods. It is food that has been created artificially by a corporation or a company whose primary purpose is to make a profit, not to make us healthier. Some examples are orange juice, canned syrups, frozen dinners, bread, yogurts and cereals. In all of these products, different natural foods are taken, processed, mixed, combined with unnatural fats and/or unnatural carbohydrates, chemicals, flavor enhancers, color additives and other chemicals like preservatives, and then packaged and sent to the market. They taste delicious and they provide enjoyment, but because of their omega-6s they also stimulate a chronic inflammatory response that leads to disease. Yes, besides increasing your weight and pushing you closer to diabetes, ultimately these products will make you ill.

Processed foods are divided into three main groups:

1. **Fatty foods:** foods containing processed fat and vegetable oils. Processed fats are known as trans fatty acids: man-made fats that do not become rancid and are excellent for preservation. They are found in all kinds of packaged and canned foods. The problem is that both the trans fatty acids and vegetable oils are high in omega-6s, which means they are pro-inflammatory and toxic. Examples of these fatty processed foods are cheeses, spreads, dips, sauces, snacks, soups, frozen meals, cookies, hot dogs, muffins, etc.

2. **Carbohydrate-containing foods.** Processed carbohydrates are carbohydrate-containing foods that have gone through a manufacturing process; their structures are broken-down, manipulated, cooked and simplified ("pre-digested") for ease of eating. Once eaten, they are absorbed quickly by the body, stimulating the omega-6 system and the production of insulin. In their original, unprocessed state, these foods could be good sources of omega-3s. But processing puts them on the omega-6 pathway where they become "foods" that cause obesity, inflammation and diseases such as diabetes. Examples of this include tomato juice (from tomatoes), apple juice and apple jelly (from apples), orange juice, orange jelly and orange marmalade (from oranges), flour products, pasta and breads (from flour), breakfast cereals (from grains), grape juice and grape jelly (from grapes), potato chips and mashed potatoes (from potatoes); corn muffins, corn chips and corn tortillas (from corn). Also included in this group are beer, rice cakes, donuts and sherbets.

   Processed carbohydrates are omega-6 activators.

3. **Combination foods.** Food containing processed carbohydrates and processed fats represent our food industry at its worst. Food manufacturers' extremely successful effort to generate highly durable foods with longer shelf lives has created a toxic mess for the human body. This is evidenced by escalating rates of diabetes and other Occidental diseases like cancer. These combinations are packaged breads, cakes, frozen dinners, yogurt, candy bars, chocolate milk, bakery products, ice cream, cookies, canned meals, canned soups, canned pasta, etc.

   Vegetable oils, trans fatty acids (synthetic fat) and processed carbohydrates are the lifeblood of the food industry but, sadly, at the root of our increasingly diseased society.

FATS: THE BAD AND THE GOOD

Another important food category to avoid occurs in both processed and unprocessed foods: saturated fat. This is the fat that comes from animals, especially from red meat. It is found mainly in beef, pork, veal, burgers, meat products, cold cuts, deli meat, sausage, salami, bacon, pâté and also in the fat of chicken and turkey and all products cooked with lard or animal fats. Saturated fat tastes good, especially when fried or grilled.

We humans have a pleasure center for fat, and foods fried with fat. Nathan Pritikin described this very well in his books, and I recommend that you read them if you want to learn more about this issue. Apparently, as part of the evolution of primitive man, our ancestors developed a "fat instinct center" somewhere in the brain. This center, which is strongly associated with our instinct for preservation, caused primitive and non-primitive humans to gorge on fat whenever possible.

Gorging on fat was a survival technique, providing people with large amounts of calories that would help them survive until the next time food became available. Since food was not readily available in those times, people whose brains had a well-developed "pleasure center" for the taste of fat survived through natural selection; those without this center would perish in the face of drought, famine, disease, frigid weather and similar adversities. All of us, therefore, are descendants of those who survived. We all have this fat instinct in us, some more, some less.

You experience the awakening of your fat instinct, for example, when you become hungry while driving past a hamburger place. You can also feel it when you get an uncontrollable desire to eat meat. Although in old times, the generous consumption of meat, meat products, pork, organ meats, etc., was nutritionally important, nowadays it is no longer so. You should forget about how important this type of food was in the 18th century when the American colonies were fighting England, or in Europe 500 years ago, or now for struggling communities in Africa, and understand that the meat products that we mention here give you two bad things: saturated fat that clogs your blood vessels and coronary arteries, and excessive amounts of omega-6 fatty acids, which give you bad eicosanoids and excessive inflammation.

Unfortunately, it gets worse. The pleasure center related to this fat instinct frequently wants to be satisfied, and can easily control a person. Fortunately, this does not happen to every human being, as the center is not the same for everybody. It is strong in some people while weak in others. But those with even a mild urge for fat do get the call for meat and other fatty foods. You can see them filling the steakhouses, hamburger places and restaurants. You see them buying meat products, you hear them when they describe with pride how their freezer is full of meat. It is the same in every country – only the type of meat product varies.

So, now that you understand this, you can see the conflict: the instinct of your body will call you to consume foods containing saturated fat, even though this kind of food actually hurts you.

Consumption of foods containing saturated fat is without any doubt a source of health problems and should be restricted in everyone's diet, and particularly for those suffering from arthritis, inflammatory diseases, pains and injuries.

The three bad fats

Reviewing the above, the three bad fats with omega-6s are:

1. Saturated fat, which is the fat from animal products we've just described.

2. Fried foods or foods cooked with oil or fat.

3. Trans fatty acids or processed fat contained in processed foods.

The good fat

The good fats provide helpful omega-3s. This is the fat in fish, especially oily fish such as salmon, trout, tuna, cod, sardines, anchovies, bluefish and mackerel. It also comes in olive oil, olives, flaxseeds, flaxseed oil, avocados, walnuts, and walnut oil.

AVOID OMEGA-6

Foods containing omega-6 fatty acids and those that activate the toxic omega-6 metabolic pathway should be avoided.

Sources of omega-6s:

- Meat and meat products (especially red meat: pork, beef, lamb, and veal)
- Dairy products
- Poultry
- Sesame oil
- Corn
- Peanuts, peanut oil and peanut butter
- Vegetable oil (soybean, safflower, sunflower, corn, and cotton seed)
- The three bad fats: saturated fats from animal products, fat from fried food, and trans fatty acids from processed food

Activators of toxic omega-6s:

- Deficit of antioxidants (excess of free radicals)
- Excessive alcohol consumption
- Excessive quantities of coffee and sugar
- Flour products (bread, pasta, cakes, pastry, donuts, bagels and bakery products)
- Fruit juices
- High simple-carbohydrate diets
- Processed carbohydrates (simple carbohydrates)
- Stress
- Uncontrolled diabetes

Let me give you some examples. Pork lo mein with a beer and dessert, or pasta and meatballs with a couple of beers are all omega-6 meals. Chicken fried with corn oil, rice cakes with peanut butter, a breakfast with orange juice, cereal and fat-free milk are all examples of omega-6 meals. Working under stress while drinking plenty of coffee and snacking on donuts and cake, or enjoying football on Sunday with lots of beer, chips and dips are omega-6 activators. A large hamburger with fries, a large steak with mashed potatoes, a typical Mexican meal, a large pastrami sandwich, a couple of cocktails with some peanuts, fettuccine Alfredo, or bagels with cream cheese are all omega-6 activators. They all push you deeper into the pro-inflammatory omega-6/free-radical state that, when chronic, shows up as ongoing disease, including pain and inflammation.

CHOLESTEROL AND CRP

To lower levels of cholesterol and LDL, the bad cholesterol

It is very simple. To lower cholesterol and LDLs (low-density lipoprotein), avoid omega-6 foods and follow the Mediterranean Diet. Nevertheless, you may have a congenital tendency to have high cholesterol. If this dietary program does not work to reduce your cholesterol in six weeks, you may need a dietary adjustment, and if that does not work, you may need medications. See your doctor in this case.

To raise levels HDL, the good cholesterol

HDL, or high-density lipoprotein, is the good cholesterol and works as a detergent, cleaning the pipes (arteries and coronaries). The higher the HDLs the better, since it prevents coronary disease, heart attacks and strokes.

These are the recommendations to increase HDL:

- Regular exercise
- Nuts (mainly walnuts but also macadamias and pumpkin seeds; on occasion some almonds and hazelnuts)
- Olives, black or green
- Olive oil – at least one or two large tablespoons twice a day
- Mediterranean Diet
- Fish (mainly oily fish like anchovies, bluefish, cod, halibut, mackerel, salmon, sardines, trout and tuna)
- Fish-oil gel caps, salmon-oil gel caps, or cod liver oil
- Ground flaxseeds and flaxseed oil, liquid or gel caps
- Omega-3 foods, such as algae and green leafy vegetables (alfalfa sprouts, arugula, broccoli, cauliflower, collard greens, kale, lettuce, mustard greens, romaine, spinach and watercress)

To lower levels of CRP

C-reactive protein (CRP) is a marker for inflammation in the body, detected by a blood test. When elevated, it is an indicator of active inflammation and ongoing disease, or threat of disease. Just as lava can erupt from a volcano anywhere on Earth, this inflammation may erupt anywhere in the body and may explode as colitis, heart attack, arthritis, or an injury that does not heal. It may also erupt as pain, severe atherosclerosis, lack of immunity and many other metabolic disorders.

These are the recommendations to lower CRP levels:

- Decrease omega-6 intake
- Increase omega-3 intake
- Get antioxidants, from either fresh foods (fruits, vegetables, herbs) or supplements
- If taking omega-3 supplements (fish oil, salmon oil) vitamins

and antioxidant pills, take only the recommended brands and avoid unreliable brands

- Avoid the three bad fats
- Consider taking supplements of GLA (gamma-linoleic acid). See Chapter 9 for more information, or ask your doctor about it
- Control diabetes, infections and dental diseases
- Follow the Mediterranean Diet
- Take olive oil twice a day

A FEW THINGS TO REMEMBER

→ **Beef eaters don't last long.**

→ **Fat-free diets are dangerous; everyone needs good fats.**

→ **If omega-3 pushes your car to the west and omega-6 pushes your car to the east, you may not get anywhere.**

→ **The poker game called your life may depend on your essential fatty acid cards: Too many sixes and just a few threes and you lose, but plenty of threes and only a few sixes and you win. Some people cheat and win, but most of those who cheat lose it all. Do you want to gamble with your life?**

THE ANTI-NUTRIENT LIFESTYLE

Joints, heart, muscles, coronary arteries and all the organs of the body are made of living tissue, fibers, cells and complex proteins. Daily use causes wear and tear, and demands a daily supply of nutrients to help with the repair. A smoker who abuses alcohol, for example, lives in a state of permanent physical stress. As such, his or her system will contain excessive amounts of free radicals. In the absence of adequate nutrition from fresh fruits and vegetables, omega-3 fatty acids, proper protein, vitamins and minerals, the excessive free radicals will not be neutralized by antioxidants and tissue damage will occur. Additionally, if such a person eats too much saturated fat, and high amounts of sugars and flour products, dairy products, meat, potatoes, fried food, fast food, frozen dinners, processed foods, processed fats, vegetable oils and juices (which are all factory or man-made foods instead of natural food), his or her diet would be full of the harmful omega-6 fatty acids, which generate bad eicosanoids. Even if this person eats a lot of food, he or she will be nutritionally deficient because there are few good nutrients in these foods. This is essentially an anti-nutrient diet, and is damaging to the heart, joints, coronary arteries, cartilage, ligaments, muscle, and all the organs of the body.

A person following this anti-nutrient diet is full of free radicals and bad eicosanoids, which cause tissue damage, promote inflammation and arthritis, and favor heart trouble in the form of coronary disease and atherosclerosis.

The situation worsens when the person is affected by the chemicals and additives found in these foods, processed meats and soft drinks. Corn, corn products, fast food (like hamburgers, pizza and hot dogs), peanuts, peanut butter, vegetable oil, fatty snacks, fatty dips and dressings are particularly high in omega-6s, generating even more bad eicosanoids (bad prostaglandins) and inflammation.

If you thought that meat and potatoes, orange juice, cheeseburgers, a bagel with cream cheese, cereal with milk, the milk you see in the commercial ("Got Milk?"), salad dressings, and the chips and dips consumed during Sunday's televised sports programs were any good for you, think again! They are all omega-6 foods, promoting arthritis and pain. They are also enemies of the heart. Like beer, bakery products, cookies and cream, they are all pro-inflammatories.

If all of this was not enough, certain kinds of foods create more acidity in the body making the damage to the tissues even worse. These foods are alcohol, cheeses, cocoa, corn and corn products, coffee, flour products, pasta, meat, sugar, sugar products (e.g. candies, pastries, and snacks), vinegar, peanuts and peanut butter. These foods create acidity that will attack the organs and tissues of our bodies, doubling their adverse effects on tissues. Hence, they should be eliminated from the diet.

More poor food choices (because of their omega-6 content) are cakes, canned creamy soups, donuts, fried food, frozen meals, margarine, mayonnaise, canned food with fat, bakery products (muffins, bagels, bread, pastries, cookies), chips, dips, take-out food, packaged bread, waffles, processed meat products (salami, hot dogs, pepperoni, bologna, etc.).

PRO-INFLAMMATORY FOODS

Certain foods are pro-inflammatory because they create acidity in the tissues, have excessive omega-6s, lack omega-3s or antioxidants, or any and all of these reasons. While I've mentioned them before, these pro-inflammatory foods need to be mentioned again:

Foods with high levels of omega-6 (also known as linoleic acid) such as red meat (from pork, beef, lamb and veal), chicken, turkey, vegetable oils (corn oil, safflower, sunflower, peanut, cottonseed and soy oil) as well as the oils in processed and packaged food. This group also includes peanuts and peanut butter, cashews and pecans, and sunflower and sesame seeds. Foods cooked in peanut, sesame and sunflower oils, such as restaurant food, ethnic food, fried food and fast food are considered pro-inflammatory.

Saturated fat that comes from animal fat, dairy products, butter and tropical oils.

Trans fatty acids, which are man-made (factory-made) fats, found in processed foods, salad dressings, margarine, bakery products (cookies, bread, muffins, bagels, donuts, crackers, etc.), salsa and dips.

Pulses such as green peas, chickpeas and corn that also have omega-6.

Processed carbohydrates such as flour products, sugars, sweet drinks and juices, candies, snacks, dips, all bakery products, pasta, cereal, breakfast cereal, alcohol (beer, liquor). They all stimulate the omega-6 pathway as well.

Fast foods, including fried food and culturally specific food, are particularly bad because they contain heavy amounts of the items listed above. These foods often combine processed carbohydrates with fried vegetable oil, meat, animal fat or grains with trans fatty acid and fried vegetable oil. Fast foods are anti-nutrient foods and, perhaps, the worst. They owe this dubious honor to the fact that they combine two of the worst offenders – processed carbohydrates and heated oil in the form of fried foods.

Fried food. The worst kind of food is food cooked in oil that is re-used, commonly found at state fairs, hamburger restaurants, fast-food restaurants, street food vendors, etc.

Certain conditions generate free radicals and bad eicosanoids: smoking, exposure to pollutants and chemicals, stress, excessive caffeine consumption, viral and bacterial infections, obesity and diabetes.

AN ANTI-INFLAMMATORY DIET

The Jupiter Institute Omega Diet is a program rich in omega-3 fatty acids, which are natural anti-inflammatory nutrients. They come from fish, fish products, fish oil, flaxseed, certain nuts, supplements and vegetables. The diet provides olive oil, well known for its anti-inflammatory properties, and also fresh herbs, fruits and vegetables known for their powerful antioxidant effect. Antioxidants are seriously important because they neutralize those unhealthy free radicals that cause so much harm to the injured tissue.

One of our program's goals is to disengage the person from the food that provides omega-6 fatty acids, which causes inflammation in joints, tendons, muscles, and the other tissues and organs of the body. Just increasing the intake of the good omega-3s, however, is not enough. The intake of omega-6s needs to be decreased. If you have just eaten corn with margarine and fried chicken, you cannot fix it by having some spinach and olive oil when you get home. A few capsules of salmon oil can't erase the adverse effects of two cheeseburgers with French fries. If you want to enjoy the benefits of the program and avoid the damaging effect of anti-nutrients, you must increase the intake of foods containing omega-3s while decreasing or altogether avoiding the intake of omega-6 foods. I'll say it again: you can't expect to feast on pizza and cake or French fries and beer and then come home and clean up your act by taking two tablespoons of olive oil and a few gel caps of salmon oil.

INFLAMMATION: THE "MOTHER OF ALL DISEASES"?

We now have good evidence of a common link between the origins of heart disease, arthritis, stroke, cancer and many other ailments. It is the chronic inflammation caused by poor nutrition that triggers the toxic omega-6/free-radical state in the body.

Research shows that an advanced omega-6/free-radical state induces atherosclerosis and the slow closing of the coronaries, decreasing blood flow to the heart. This encourages the development of coronary artery disease, which can lead to angina, heart attack and even sudden cardiac death. This same toxic state creates pro-inflammatory compounds that attack the joints, hurt the cartilage and ligaments, decreasing repair and inducing osteoarthritis.

In an injured person, this inflammatory state will hamper healing. An excess of omega-6 fatty acids and free radicals produces arthritis and interferes with the healing of joints and injuries, and, therefore, increases the need for pharmaceutical drugs and doctor visits.

This inflammatory state increases the risk for stroke and cancer and decreases the ability of the cells be healthy and to repair themselves. Other disorders caused by the inflammatory, omega-6/ free-radical state are diabetes, and mental health diseases such as depression and other psychiatric disorders. This omega-6/free-radical state is a common link, a common root, a common source of all the diseases we mentioned above – heart disease, coronary disease, joint disease, musculoskeletal diseases and many, many organ disorders.

How can all these conditions be linked to a single cause? Imagine the body is the Earth and the inflammatory state is the lava, kept under pressure somewhere at the core of the planet. Time goes by, and the pressure of the lava grows. It may take an unpredictable amount of time but, for sure, one day that lava will burst out. The day this happens, the volcano may erupt anywhere. It may erupt in Iowa or Italy, in Mexico, China or Portugal.

Somehow, somewhere, the lava's pressure will cause an eruption. This is the same way that inflammation builds in our body, and it can erupt in the joints, in the heart, in the brain or in the prostate. It may be a long, slow eruption, like fatigue, depression, headaches and backaches, or a brutal sudden eruption such as acute colitis, heart attack or acute arthritis, or worse.

Although volcanoes appear at different times and have different strengths, the damage they cause varies widely. The common link in all these events is the pressure of the lava. The same thing happens in our body with inflammation.

Although arthritis, stroke, colitis, pains and digestive problems appear to have no link, they, in fact, do. The chronic inflammatory state (the omega-6/free-radical state) is the link. Studies confirm that if the ratio of omega-3 to omega-6 improves, the biology of the body improves. If the intake of omega-6 decreases significantly, free radicals are neutralized with antioxidants, and the intake of omega-3 foods and fish oils expands, then healing increases and diseases are either slowed or prevented.

REVIEW: ANTI-INFLAMMATORY FOODS

The anti-inflammatory foods are:

Foods that provide omega-3 fatty acids:

- Cold-water fish (anchovies, bluefish, cod, halibut, herring, salmon, sardines, trout, and tuna).

- Green, leafy vegetables, such as arugula, broccoli, collard greens, kale, herbs (such as mint), lettuce, mustard greens, spinach, Swiss chard, and watercress.

- Nuts and seeds containing omega-3s, such as walnuts, flaxseeds and flaxseed oil, macadamias, and occasionally almonds and hazelnuts.

- Chicken and eggs enriched with omega-3.

Foods combining omega-3s and omega-9s

- Olives

- Olive oil

- Avocados

- Macadamia nuts

Foods high in antioxidants (found in fresh and dried herbs, fresh fruits and vegetables, and red wine)

- Vitamins A, C, E and the B-vitamins

- Minerals such as selenium, copper and zinc

- GLA (gamma-linoleic acid – found in borage seed oil, evening primrose oil and black-currant oil)

TAKING PRACTICAL STEPS TO CHANGE YOUR DIET

Here are a few guidelines and hints to help you put into practice all the theories you have read in the preceding pages.

• Reduce the amount of processed food in your diet and add fresh, natural food.

• Eat more fish, especially fish that contains omega-3s.

• Buy eggs labeled omega-3 or free-range.

• Buy chicken and beef from free-range or grass-fed animals.

• Make a colorful salad by using several vegetables of different kinds.

• Consume dry seasonings and plenty of fresh herbs; add them to your meals every day.

• Plan your meals ahead of time so you avoid the wrong foods.

• Olive oil and olives contain the good omega oil. Eat a lot of them; they are good for you. However, corn, peanuts, sunflower, soybeans, safflower and cottonseed oils have too much omega-6, which is bad for you and you need to avoid them. Some authors favor canola oil, which contains both omega-6 and omega-3. However, its refining process produces impurities – certain compounds that make it undesirable for consumption. Walnut oil is okay.

• Vegetable oils and vegetable shortening, butter, margarine and salad dressings that are not fat-free are not allowed. On the other hand, walnuts and flaxseeds are excellent sources of omega-3s and you should feel free to consume them.

- Avoid sugar and sugared drinks, sodas, soft drinks, commercial fruit juices. Avoid candies, sweets and desserts. Energy drinks and the so-called thirst quenchers are not at all OK.

- Reduce your consumption of flour products such as bread, pasta, cookies and bakery products.

- In general, avoid dairy products. It is okay to have some milk in your morning coffee, a bit of sour cream or yogurt a couple of times a week, but no more than that. (Half-and-half and nondairy creamers are nothing but gross nutritional mistakes.) It is OK to have small amounts of fat-free cheeses or cottage cheese.

- Fast foods, whether eaten in fast-food places, restaurants, or at home are not advised. Just because you prepare your own hamburgers, pizza or tacos does not make these foods good for you. They are still unhealthy for the body. So, ban pizza, pasta, mozzarella, hamburgers, French fries, fried chicken and hot dogs from your diet.

- When you crave snacks, eat olives, fruits and nuts, especially walnuts. Walnuts and pumpkin seeds are first-place finishers in that race. Almonds and hazelnuts are in second place. All the other nuts are in third place, except for peanuts and pecans, which are in not in the race at all!

- Stay away from pro-inflammatory foods. Omega-6 foods, such as vegetable oils, fried food, processed food, all fast food, packaged food, prepared food, packaged snacks prepared with sugar, most salad dressings, bread and bakery products and most packaged microwave foods should be avoided. The same is true for trans fatty acids like salad dressings, processed cheeses, processed sauces, dips, packaged food, frozen dinners, food made with shortening or margarine, cakes, and cookies.

• Avoid the "omega-6/free-radical state" discussed earlier. Free radicals occur constantly, even if you live a normal life, with normal metabolism. In addition, smoking, alcohol, drugs, processed food, anti-nutritious food, pollutants, bad fats and stress all generate more free radicals. The free radicals interfere with the omega fatty acid metabolism, and they attack the good omega-3s, causing tissue damage and inflammation. Avoiding all the things mentioned above decreases the amount of free radicals, giving the antioxidants a better chance at neutralizing them. Antioxidants are your daily antibody against free radicals; they are very good for you. The best antioxidants come from nature – fresh fruits, fresh vegetables and fresh herbs. Eat them! You can also increase your intake of antioxidants by taking supplements: see Chapter 9.

• Red wine is allowed and encouraged in our program, in small to moderate amounts. It is the only alcohol you are allowed to have. Never have more than 4 ounces a day and always with lunch or dinner, and not earlier.

Pay Attention to the Ratio Of Omega-3 to Omega-6

You should focus your diet on food that provides omega-3 and antioxidants. When you eat a typical American diet, you get large amounts of omega-6s and very few omega-3s (sometimes the relationship between the bad omega-6s and the good omega-3s is as high as 30 or 40 to 1). Two things happen as a result: the excessive amount of omega-6 neutralizes what few omega-3s are in the diet, and whatever omega-3s are left will be attacked by free radicals. The end result is that you will have a final ratio of omega-6 to omega-3 sometimes as high as 60:1 or 80:1! This keeps you in a "pro-inflammatory"' omega-6/free radical state.

So, even if you modify your diet to include good sources of omega-3s (adding olive oil to a salad, or eating salmon or walnuts every once in a while, for example), until you do something to decrease free radicals and the abuse of omega-6 foods, your omega-3s will be neutralized. Keep in mind that omega-3s and omega-6s compete, so the body cannot use omega-3s efficiently if there are too many omega-6s in the body, and if this happens, the pathway of good eicosanoids is blocked.

However, you can change that. If you eat your chicken with olive oil on a bed of colorful salad and have fresh fruit for dessert, you will be changing the ratio – you will be getting fewer omega-6s and more omega-3s and protective antioxidants. This will lower your ratio of omega-6 to omega-3 to 10:1, and if you exchange the chicken for salmon it may end up with a very beneficial ratio of 5:1, which is excellent. As another example, if you change your breakfast to consuming omega-3 eggs with a bit of olive oil instead of cereal with milk, or bread with jelly and peanut butter, you are changing the omega-6 to omega-3 ratio. If you are accustomed to eating your pasta with sauce or meatballs, eat it instead with olive oil and fresh herbs, accompanied by a salad; again, you will be making the omega-6 to omega-3 ratio more beneficial.

Remember what I said earlier: eating omega-3 foods alone is not enough. You need to lower your intake of omega-6 foods in order for the ratio to improve significantly. You also need to avoid the foods, drinks and situations that trigger free radicals, and you need to increase your intake of antioxidants. Decreasing free radicals and increasing antioxidants will protect your omega-3s. If you change your cocktails and peanuts for red wine and olives, you would have an improvement to your omega ratio. Exchanging a hamburger and French fries for grilled beef over a bed of salad, and trading in your barbecued chicken with lots of mashed potatoes for half that chicken with rice and beans and olive oil also improves your ratio. I will return to this subject in Chapter 11 and show you how to prepare some "Mediterraneanized" dishes.

By following the Jupiter Institute Omega Diet, you will consume omega-3 foods and antioxidants and avoid omega-6 foods. The Jupiter Institute Omega Diet is basically an improved Mediterranean Diet, enhanced with certain modifications and additions described earlier.

The Mediterranean Diet is a fascinating field to explore. Not only do grain and protein sources vary from country to country, but so do wonderful spices and seasonings. We invite you to learn more by visiting your library and local bookstores. Check our website (www.jupiterinstitute.com) to find the books we read and recommend regarding this diet.

CHAPTER EIGHT

Why Alternative Therapies Are Effective

Have no doubt: alternative medicine therapies are very effective. We use them in our Jupiter Institute Pain Program for one simple reason: they work. We explain to our patients and readers how integrating them with conventional medicine provides relief and enhances repair in individuals suffering from pain, arthritis and injuries.

Alternative medicine offers patients another avenue to gain control of their disease. Millions of people suffering from pain, arthritis and injuries have embraced alternative therapies with excellent results. Although not successful in every case, alternative medicine offers us a chance to find relief from ailments without having to deal with the negative aspects of pharmaceutical drugs (and their side effects) and surgeries so commonplace in conventional medicine.

I want to emphasize, however, that there is no substitute for conventional medicine in the case of a great many health conditions. Alternative medicine should not replace proven medical treatments. As much as we may support and encourage alternative medicine, in cases of sepsis (infections), fractures, surgical conditions, heart attacks, pneumonia, heart disease, bleeding, strokes and many other acute or chronic diseases, conventional medicine cannot be replaced. Hundreds of diseases of the eyes, ears, nose, throat, chest and abdomen can only be taken care of by what is still one of the most wonderful advancements of mankind: conventional medicine.

In truth, there is no substitution for individuals taking care of themselves, and making a healthy, inflammation-free lifestyle – as outlined in this book – a priority. This would go a long way toward preventing many of the diseases affecting millions of people in America today.

Nevertheless, there has been and continues to be a growing dissatisfaction with conventional medicine. Many call this healthcare system impersonal because doctors practice a medicine influenced by attorneys and pharmaceutical companies. Many also call it ineffective due to its lack of success in treating the chronic conditions plaguing us today, including lifestyle diseases such as cancer, arthritis, diabetes, obesity and heart disease. The invasion of HMOs, the ever-increasing price of health insurance and the growing disappointments on the part of both doctors and patients have only made matters worse. Citizens (including healthcare professionals) lament that the overall quality of medical care has been decreasing over the past several years and that the government and major medical companies have done nothing to fix it. Faced with these real problems – and in light of the positive findings related to alternative therapies – a growing number of patients find it hard to accept that most doctors do not recognize the benefit of alternative medicine.

These disappointments have created a fertile ground for alternative medical therapies, which have been growing steadily in the U.S. for years. People began looking into alternative therapies and discovered that in many cases the practitioner is usually a very pleasant person (unlike many doctors), and treatment is mostly comfortable and effective. Friends told their neighbors and relatives. As the news got passed on, the popularity of these therapies spread throughout the country, and even more studies are being conducted now to support their efficacy.

The fact is that Americans are finding relief in alternative medicine that they often cannot find in conventional medicine. Whether used alone or in combination with mainstream medicine or other conventional therapies, alternative medicine offers tools and remedies that work. It provides relief from pain and other symptoms of conditions like arthritis while providing overall health benefits.

Most people suffering from pain, arthritis and injuries consult a physician first. This is still the best initial path, since a combination of prescription medications (NSAIDs, pain medications, etc.), physical therapy and sometimes a cortisone injection may provide significant relief from acute conditions, while providing time to investigate the root causes of the disorder.

In a few cases, this initial treatment may provide permanent relief. In the majority of cases, however, symptoms and conditions persist, particularly if the person is not consuming a Mediterranean-style Diet. This is a true "crossroads" – the right time to stop, think and consider how alternative medicine can help.

Both physician and patient may choose to continue on the conventional path, even after X-rays, lab tests, an MRI and an accurate diagnosis show that there are no major lesions or pathological disorders. On this path, after one, two or three trials of medications, injections or physical therapy, patients will be sent to specialists for more therapy, medications, nerve conduction studies, another MRI, perhaps, and additional lab tests. While this could be the right path for some patients, it often brings more suffering. Subjecting a person to strong medication, unnecessary injections, excessively lengthy therapy and a surfeit of tests can cause tremendous stress. All too frequently they lose hope of ever being cured. Many people who follow this path find themselves losing their independence and sometimes even their jobs and relationships. They bounce from one doctor to the next – without relief – and end up drowning themselves in a sea of narcotics. It is for these reasons that I created the Jupiter Institute Program.

There is another choice at the crossroads. Both patient and doctor can acknowledge the value of alternative therapies, and that the condition will likely have a better chance for improvement by including them. At this point (generally the second or third visit), the doctor who is considering additional medications and conventional treatments, should also contemplate integrating alternative therapies such as chiropractic care, acupuncture, and nutritional adjustment. Treatment protocols can be discussed between patient and doctor, and experts brought in as necessary. There is enough scientific proof for the success of alternative therapies to support and encourage this option. My message to patients and doctors alike is this: yes, there is another option – a new and extremely positive one – that is showing consistent promise and success. These therapists are not in competition with doctors or other therapists, and they can be extremely effective in helping doctors get their patients better, sooner.

The problem that might arise is that there may not be a center like ours near you that will provide integrated treatment protocols. Practitioners of alternative medicine therapies may be scattered throughout your area or even in another town. The best advice in this case is to do what you can. Find high-quality alternative therapy practitioners in your local area and visit them. (Health food stores are generally a good resource.) Ask them how they would treat your condition and, if you feel comfortable, try their treatment. Chiropractors, acupuncturists, reflexologists, physical therapists and nutritionists can be helpful in establishing an effective treatment program for pain conditions, as well as a myriad of other diseases and illnesses. Many of these consultants will be happy to share 10 minutes of their time to tell you what they do. Some may even provide a treatment for no charge.

ALTERNATIVE THERAPIES THAT CAN HELP ARTHRITIS AND OTHER PAINFUL CONDITIONS

Alternative therapies are a group of different treatment modalities, developed in different countries and supported by extensive experience. Not all alternative therapies are indicated for arthritis, pain and injuries.

Here are some of the most highly recommended forms of alternative medicine that provide benefits in the treatment of arthritis, pain, injuries, neck and back pain, muscle and tendon pain, bursitis and fatigue:

• Nutrition therapy
• Acupuncture
• Chiropractic care
• Nutritional supplements
• Tai chi
• Reflexology
• Therapeutic massage
• Acupressure

Some other forms of alternative medicine may provide additional benefit to individuals suffering from these conditions as well as other illnesses and may improve their general well-being. These therapies are:

• Alexander technique
• Herbal medicine
• Ayurvedic medicine
• Qi gong
• Homeopathy
• Craniosacral therapy
• Meditation
• Reiki
• Yoga

We urge you to learn about these therapies as you may find significant relief, healing, and reduction of distress in one or more of them.

I have found the book *Clinicians' Complete Reference to Complementary and Alternative Medicine* by Donald Novey, M.D. (Published by Mosby) to be an excellent reference.

Official Recognition

In response to the growth of alternative and integrative medicine, the government created the White House Commission on Complementary and Alternative Medicine (WHCCAM). Its purpose is to study and evaluate alternative therapies and the effectiveness of complementary medical programs. This commission evaluated the data published in journals and books, and listened to statements from professors, lay people, physicians, scientists, patients and practitioners. The conclusion was clear: alternative medicine was found to be very effective for the management of pain, arthritis and injuries. Accordingly, the commission created the National Center for Complementary and Alternative Medicine, acknowledging alternative and integrative medicine as part of a complete health care delivery system. You are welcome to visit this site at the National Institutes of Health (www.nih.gov).

The Jupiter Institute Pain Program

I chose to integrate three of the most important alternative medicine therapies into our pain-relief program: acupuncture, chiropractic care, and nutritional supplements. The first two are discussed below, the last in Chapter 9. I chose the first two because they have proven to be consistently helpful in alleviating pain, and the third because nutrition is a core consideration for eliminating and avoiding pain conditions.

Our program integrates these three therapies with four others: conventional internal medicine care; dietary adjustment (our modified version of the Mediterranean Diet, the Jupiter Institute Omega Diet, discussed in Chapter 7); physical therapy; and exercise counseling, for a total of seven therapies. These therapies are used differently depending on the condition of the individual. We do not recommend all seven treatments for each patient, and each treatment is given with varying intensities and frequency according to the patient's needs.

You can visit our center online at www.jupiterinstitute.com. We hope our initiatives in this area will give doctors in other areas the inspiration to create similar programs for their communities. Going beyond the orthodox boundaries of conventional medicine is wise and it pays because it prioritizes the common goal: to heal.

We invite patients in other states to look for integrative medical centers such as ours. If they are not available, contact a local health professional with the reputation of being open minded to coordinated care and management. We also invite patients and physicians to read some of the excellent books mentioned on our website.

RECOMMENDATIONS

Follow these steps when considering alternative medicine or integrative medicine:

Make an informed decision. Get information from local bookstores, libraries and the internet. Ask around. Contact the professional organizations we post at the end of this book and on our website.

Use common sense. Unconventional therapies are remedies that may or may not be successful; weigh the risks and benefits. Ask your doctor to assist you as you explore other alternatives to your treatment plan.

Do not expect a miracle cure. Integrative medicine may provide relief but, like conventional medicine, may not cure the condition. Have realistic expectations and patience.

Get an accurate diagnosis. Make sure you know from your physician what type of conditions you have, so you know what you are treating.

Don't hesitate to ask questions. Ask questions like whether and how a particular therapy will help your condition.

Check references. Talk to others who have similar conditions and have gone through the same treatment.

Be suspicious if the practitioner cannot show you a professional license, asks you to stop your medications, promises you a cure or tells you not to tell your doctor.

Even if you pursue alternative medicine for your conditions, do not neglect conventional medicine therapies if you need them. You might have a condition that requires prompt medical care by a physician, and you must act on it.

ACUPUNCTURE

Acupuncture is a powerful medical technique that helps strengthen the immune system, reduce inflammation, control pain and improve the quality of life. Acupuncture is highly effective in the healing of injuries and the treatment of multiple painful conditions. Because it affects a person's inner bioenergetics, those who receive acupuncture not only heal physically but quite often experience new and profound states of peace, clarity and harmony.

It has been determined that the human body is a bioenergetic system. When this system is disturbed, pain or illness sets in. Acupuncture treatment restores energetic balance by stimulating the body's natural ability to heal itself without the use of drugs or surgery.

History

Acupuncture is one of the oldest known forms of medicine. It developed in China over 3,000 years ago, where it was used to maintain health and treat disease. Acupuncture was brought to Europe in the late 17th century and from there it has spread to other countries, including the United States. When China opened its doors in the 1970s, Americans were able to gain more direct exposure to this healing technique.

Although the American public quickly became enthusiastic about acupuncture's potential for treatment of pain and disease, American physicians were reluctant to endorse it. Even now, many American doctors refuse to accept it as a viable form of medical care. There are two reasons for this attitude. First, it has been difficult for some doctors to accept the underlying principle of acupuncture: that health and disease is directly related to the flow of energy (Qi) through the body's energetic channels (meridians). Energy medicine, although gaining popularity in Western cultures today, is not described in classic anatomy books. Secondly, attempts by American physicians to replicate the Chinese technique by practicing acupuncture themselves proved mostly unsuccessful.

For many Western doctors, acupuncture is still too new, too untraditional and too difficult to understand and practice. Nevertheless, the medical establishment's initial skepticism began to moderate in the early 1980s. Numerous articles in medical journals and books on acupuncture demonstrate its effectiveness, including its success in the treatment of pain conditions.

Currently, acupuncture is used to treat hundreds of millions of people around the world for almost every disease. It is documented that more than 15 million Americans have received acupuncture, mainly for pain control. Since pain is the number-one symptom affecting people with arthritis, acupuncture has been used to treat many kinds of arthritis, including osteoarthritis, fibromyalgia and rheumatoid arthritis.

Acupuncture is now being endorsed by the National Institutes of Health, by the White House Commission on Complementary and Alternative Medicine, and by many American medical organizations.

How it works

A person's life force or energy, called Qi (pronounced chi), does not remain stationary but flows constantly through channels in the body, much like rivers of water. These rivers of Qi are called meridians, and they connect inside the body to each other and with the deep organs. Acupuncture is performed using hair-thin needles that puncture the skin at specific places called acupuncture points.

The stimulation caused by the needle affects the flow of energy to a particular organ or area of the body, and can modify and correct the flow of Qi through a particular meridian. The needle works like a valve controlling the flow of water through a pipe.

There are many meridian systems in acupuncture, and each is accessed for different reasons. Also, there are about 360 basic acupuncture points on the surface of the body that have specific names and functions. In addition, there are several hundred "trigger points" that can also be stimulated with the needles.

All of these meridians, acupuncture points, and trigger points are interconnected by approximately 70 additional channels, forming a complex web of energetic activity. Using this knowledge, a skilled acupuncturist can open or close the valves of energy at the acupuncture points. They can decrease excess flow in high-energy areas, while increasing the flow of healing energy to low-pressure areas. The meridians are, however, invisible and do not correlate with the familiar anatomical charts of Western medicine.

In Chinese medicine, illness is a manifestation of the relationship between a patient's constitutional makeup and the stimulus of the environment. All illnesses and symptoms result from imbalances in quantity, distribution and flow of the vital energy called Qi.

A suffering or damaged area accumulates blood, fluids and Qi and becomes stagnant. Chinese medicine specifies that there must be movement of Qi, blood and fluids if a sick organ is to heal and return to balance. Where there is pain and injury, the flow is blocked. This blockage prevents that area from receiving oxygen-rich blood, among other things that aid healing. Acupuncture improves the flow and facilitates healing by eliminating the obstruction and relieving pressure in the area.

To define the movement, excesses, deficiencies and distribution of Qi in the body, the Chinese apply the concept of yin and yang. Yin and yang represent the expression of a dynamic equilibrium between excess and deficiency of Qi. While a yin condition is passive, inferior, chronic, cold and poorly defined, a yang condition will be bright, superior, active, hot and acute. A yang illness may present with a fever, heat and severe pain.

According to Chinese medicine, the balance of yin and yang within an individual must be in harmony. Qi must flow in the proper direction, allowing the yin and yang to be in equilibrium.

Acupuncturists first identify the balance of yin and yang, diagnosing the pattern and type of disharmony in a particular individual. Once the diagnosis is made, the acupuncturist searches for the appropriate meridians and acupuncture points on those meridians that control the flow of Qi to the problem area. Then, they insert the needles which, like valves, decrease or increase the energy flow and bring balance to the affected area.

Technique

Acupuncture needles used to be made of gold or silver, but nowadays they are made of stainless steel and are sterilized and individually packed. They are used to puncture the skin at acupuncture points, and sometimes rotated or moved for greater efficacy.

Electric stimuli are frequently used in combination with acupuncture. In these cases, short cable wires are connected to low-intensity units to deliver a fixed current to the acupuncture points and provide greater stimulation.

On other occasions, acupuncture is performed together with Moxa burning, in which a dry paste of the chopped leaves of mugwort (Artemisia vulgaris) is attached to the needles and lit. This procedure heats the handle of the needle, which transmits heat to the acupuncture points, augmenting the effectiveness of the treatment. All of these procedures are relatively painless.

On average, patients require between three and six acupuncture treatments to begin getting relief; although, the number of sessions will vary. Long-standing and complex chronic conditions might need one or two treatments a week for several weeks. New conditions may get relief after one or two sessions.

Acupuncture for pain, arthritis and injuries

Acupuncture is highly effective in treating both acute and chronic pain and injuries, and can be used alone or as a part of a comprehensive program.

The list of conditions effectively treated with acupuncture is extensive and includes:

* Acute arthritis
* Cancer pain
* Carpal tunnel syndrome
* Chronic arthritis
* Degenerative disc disease
* Fibromyalgia
* Headaches
* Joint pain
* Muscular injuries
* Myofascial pain
* Neck and back pain
* Neuropathy
* Pinched nerve
* Postherpetic neuralgia
* Sciatica
* Sports injuries
* Strain injuries
* Tennis elbow
* Trigeminal neuralgia
* Whiplash injuries

The advantages of integrating acupuncture into a comprehensive pain management program are numerous. In some cases, acupuncture by itself may resolve the pain while in others it will just reduce it. But in both cases it will assist the patient and the doctor to more successfully care for a medical condition. Whether for healing, or for facilitating healing, acupuncture's role in medicine is enormous.

Arthritis is something that acupuncturists commonly treat. There are several types of arthritis, and Chinese medicine classifies them according to their symptoms. The "wind" type moves from one joint to the next, the "damp" type is the swollen type, the "cold" type is cold to touch, the "hot" type is swollen and hot, and the "bony" type is the late-stage type.

These different types of arthritis require different acupuncture treatments and respond differently to the treatment. Although the response may vary from case to case, acupuncture provides many arthritic pain sufferers with an alternative or addition to modern arthritis therapy. Acupuncture can result in the powerful relief of pain, injury and arthritis.

"But acupuncture doesn't work!" I have heard this kind of comment on numerous occasions from people who have had a particular medical condition for many, many years. One patient, specifically, had been suffering from arthritis in her left hip for more than 25 years. She said after her second acupuncture session, "Oh, Doctor Nuchovich, I tried it, but acupuncture just doesn't work." What happens is that people expect from acupuncture the same immediate relief they can get with pills. This is an incorrect conclusion based on misinformation. If a joint has been degenerating for over 20 years, and consistently swollen, there is no way that one or two sessions of acupuncture can reverse it. Taking two Celebrex and one Darvocet, on the other hand, will provide fast relief, but no real healing. Acupuncture and pills are completely different – one is a healing technique while the other is simply a cover-up for symptoms. Acupuncture addresses the imbalance causing the pain; pills just mask the pain. Understand that it takes time for the body to erase years of abnormalities, and have patience with the healing process.

Other indications for acupuncture

Acupuncture is also used to effectively treat numerous other conditions:

Respiratory problems
- Hay fever
- Asthma
- Bronchitis
- Rhinitis
- Allergies
- Sinusitis

Neurological problems

- Facial pain
- Fatigue
- Stroke
- Paralysis
- Memory problems

Hearing problems

- Tinnitus
- Hearing disorders

Emotional problems

- Anxiety
- Depression
- Insomnia
- Nervousness

Digestive problems

- Abdominal pain
- Chronic diarrhea
- Colitis
- Constipation
- Gastritis
- Irritable Bowel Syndrome (IBS)
- Indigestion
- Nausea

Gynecological problems

- Cramps
- Hot flashes
- Infertility
- PMS
- Menopause
- Dysfunctional bleeding

Other conditions
- Addiction (smoking, alcohol, drugs)
- Chronic fatigue
- Gout
- Heel pain
- Impotence
- Incontinence
- Pain control
- Stress reduction
- Urinary disorders
- Weight control

It has been demonstrated through many books, studies and publications that acupuncture is an effective adjunct to conventional medical treatments and can be successfully employed alone or as part of a multi-disciplinary medical approach.

Acupuncture has also been used in spinal cord injuries and has been found to contribute to significant neurological and functional recoveries.

How to find an acupuncturist

Acupuncturists who are licensed and credentialed by the state are more likely to provide better care than those who are not. Although credentials do not ensure competency, they do indicate that the practitioner has met certain standards to treat patients. However, a certificate on the wall is no guarantee of expertise. We recommend selecting practitioners who have had formal training, rather than those who simply attended a few courses and seminars.

Be sure the doctor has completed a recognized acupuncture training program. Traditional Chinese Medicine (TCM) acupuncturists claim that many doctors who practice acupuncture do not have adequate training. They recommend finding a therapist who has many years of experience and who is trained in TCM.

Oriental acupuncturists, born and trained in the Far East, are considered the best. Some, like Dr. Pan-Jau Chi of our Jupiter Institute, are considered exceptional healers. A graduate of China Medical College, Dr. Chi became the medical director of the famous Keelung Acupuncture Hospital in Taiwan. After moving to the United States, he became a valued member of the Acupuncture and Oriental Medicine Alliance as well as The American Association of Oriental Medicine. He is an ideal acupuncturist.

Do not necessarily use the first acupuncturist you find; instead, search for acupuncturists in your area. When you find them, inquire about their background, their training and their experience before you consider treatment. If possible, arrange to meet with them before you commit to a session.

Acupuncture is recognized and recommended by the following organizations: The National Institutes of Health, The National Center for Complementary and Alternative Medicine (a subdivision of the US Department of Health and Human Services), The White House Commission on Complementary and Alternative Medicine, Harvard Medical School, The University of Maryland and numerous colleges and universities throughout the country.

The Arthritis Foundation and pain organizations also recognize acupuncture as a major treatment modality. Additional recommendations come from Spaulding Rehabilitation Hospital (Boston), Albert Einstein College of Medicine (New York), University of Massachusetts, Columbia University (New York), University of Arizona and many scientific publications and books.

A final note: Acupuncture offers the promise of treatment that in some cases will reduce or eliminate the need for medications and in others will ameliorate conditions for which Western medicine is unsuccessful or incomplete. Acupuncture, as a modality, is widely acknowledged as a safe procedure. In the hands of a well-trained practitioner complications are very rare.

Chiropractic Care

Chiropractic care is perhaps the most popular alternative medicine treatment in the United States. Chiropractic care treats diseases by moving and adjusting the bones of the spine and other structures. These manipulations are based on the belief that diseases are caused by pressure, especially of vertebrae and discs, on the nerves.

Doctors of chiropractic do not use drugs, injections or surgery in their practice. They also believe that the body responds to stressful conditions in a way that affects the nervous, immune and metabolic systems simultaneously. Working on the spine, for instance, may actually provide benefits to organs and metabolic systems throughout the body.

Chiropractic treatment is a wonderful technique that provides enormous relief in such conditions as arthritis, pain and injuries. Criticized by physicians who were too stubborn to investigate it, or perhaps too afraid to accept it, chiropractic treatment has survived the challenges of our modern medical society. It has proven itself as a technique that provides relief and improves quality of life, and it has saved numerous people from unnecessary surgery.

There are more than 60,000 chiropractic doctors in the United States. According to recent surveys, there has been a significant increase in the use of chiropractic health care by the general population. Chiropractors typically train for eight years prior to entering into private practice. There is an undergraduate as well as a post-graduate professional college study program as well as a clinical internship. The areas of science and clinical studies are those pertinent to the total health care of humans including anatomy, physiology, diagnosis, nutrition, pathology, radiology and therapeutics.

Doctors of chiropractic have been recognized as providing exceptional care for back pain, headaches, neck pain, nerve disorders and other spinal related conditions. In addition, chiropractors have been proponents of recognizing the capacity and integrity of body and mind to deal with stress and disease. They have collectively criticized the overuse and abuse of drugs, injections and surgery.

Chiropractic care seeks to restore normal physiologic function and thereby improve the health of the individual. The principle of treatment is based on the idea that misalignment of the vertebrae, called subluxation, causes many diseases and that chiropractic realignment of the spine is the cure. Chiropractors are trained in the highly effective technique of "unblocking" the spine, relieving its dysfunction and improving the bioelectrical conductivity of the nervous system. Chiropractic adjustments aim to restore proper spinal motion, thereby directly influencing spine-related disorders. Several publications suggest that adjustment to the spine also has the potential to influence neural (nerve) integrity, which positively affects dysfunctional organs.

For more than a century, chiropractors have advocated that an optimally functioning nervous system is necessary to good health. The significance of the nervous system and its influence on the body's ability to adapt to the environment is becoming increasingly relevant as research advances. Moreover, there is growing awareness of the need to consider prevention and health maintenance rather than waiting for disease to happen. Chiropractors typically understand this important concept, although many medical doctors do not. This is why chiropractic care is becoming a mainstream treatment for tens of millions of Americans who are seeking better health and drug-free relief.

Indications

Chiropractic treatment is recommended for the following conditions:

- Arm pain
- Arthritis
- Asthma
- Back pain
- Bursitis
- Colitis
- Cramps

- Degenerative disc disease
- Injuries
- Joint subluxation
- Menstrual cramps
- Muscle tears
- Neck pain
- Neuralgia
- Neuropathy
- Nutritional disorders
- Pinched nerve
- Respiratory disease
- Sciatica
- Tendonitis
- Tinnitus
- TMJ (temporo-mandibular joint) problems

Technique

Although chiropractors take the patient's medical history and perform a standard physical examination, it is the examination of the spine and muscle system that makes the chiropractic approach different from that of other health-care practitioners. A careful spinal examination and analysis will be performed to detect any structural abnormalities. In some cases, spinal X-rays may be necessary. The spinal examination, when analyzed through the skill and experience of a chiropractor, greatly aids in the identification of problem areas in the musculoskeletal system, which may be contributing to the ailment.

Evaluation is followed by manipulation of one or more spinal areas, and particular attention is paid to the areas of the spine where a spinal dysfunction (subluxation) has been detected. The adjustment is usually given by hand. It consists of placing the patient on a precisely designed adjustment table and then applying pressure to the areas of the spine that are out of alignment.

Doctors of chiropractic employ a wide variety of treatment methods. The experience and knowledge of the chiropractor will determine the type of manipulation and the frequency of subsequent manipulations.

Counseling

In addition to spinal manipulation, many chiropractors give nutritional advice. They also counsel on posture, on the types of sports and exercises that are best, and even on good sleeping habits. Chiropractors may recommend rehabilitative exercises and cervical support pillows. On many occasions, the treatment is complemented with physical therapy and massage to augment the healing benefits.

Counseling patients in areas such as nutrition, proper exercise and diet, lifestyle changes and general health matters demonstrates the doctor of chiropractic's concern about the "whole person."

The effectiveness of chiropractic treatment is proven by studies that demonstrate that chiropractic patients are more satisfied with their chiropractic care than with medical treatment. Chiropractic will continue to grow in this new century, and the benefits of this unique health-enhancing approach to rehabilitation will reach new levels of public awareness.

CHAPTER NINE

The Role of Supplements in Healing

 Nutritional supplements have become an essential tool in the toolbox of treatments we use to heal injuries, arthritis and pain. A good illustration of the rolethese vitamins, minerals and essential fatty acids can play in healing comes from the experience of a retired 67-year-old named James, who developed a pain between his hips and received conflicting diagnoses.

One physician told James that he had a prostate enlargement; a urologist diagnosed the pain as a hernia; and another doctor called it a pulled muscle. By the time James visited our clinic, he was confused and was taking five different medications with a range of irritating side effects. He was told that he needed surgery to correct the problem, the prospect of which was giving him nightmares.

We examined James and found a degenerative disc disease in his spine and a displaced sacrum, conditions that were affecting a nerve and producing the pain. Though James found it difficult to believe that our treatment could work without prescribed drugs, he agreed to our approach and began to work with our physical therapist and our chiropractor, who realigned his spine. Meanwhile, I put him on a daily regimen of B-complex and multiple vitamin supplements to nourish and help to repair the affected nerve.

After less than three weeks, all of James' symptoms were gone, and he was pain-free for the first time in many months. He said goodbye by coming to our clinic and leaving a bag that contained all of his medications on the counter. "Hey, doctor," he joked as he left, "You can have these. I don't need them anymore!"

No one food contains all of the vitamins and minerals that a person needs. Modern industrial farming techniques – over-cropping of the land, artificial fertilizers, early harvesting and processing of food – result in fruits and vegetables that don't have all the nutrients they should have. As a result, people need to take vitamins and other supplements in order to obtain the necessary nutrients to remain healthy. However, during illness and injury the need for those nutrients is increased. As a result, a deficiency of vitamins or minerals may affect the healing process. Moreover, if a person is on a weight-loss diet, the deficiencies may be more pronounced since typical weight-loss diets usually deprive the body of several vitamins and essential minerals. When vital nutrients are in deficit, the whole process of injury repair slows, prolonging pain and swelling as well as the suffering of affected tissues.

The United States is a country of people who are well-fed but undernourished. In general, although people eat in abundance, they do not get all the vitamins and supplements their bodies need. Some degree of vitamin and mineral deficiency is a common problem among the people of this country, and the need for supplementation is great.

As an example, a nationwide food consumption survey in 1977 and 1978 showed that more than 25% of the population was deficient in vitamin B6, vitamin A or vitamin C. The deficiency of vitamins and minerals is most pronounced in several sub-groups of the population. In addition to the chronically ill and the dieters, deficiencies were also found among adolescents, alcohol abusers, drug users, vegans, diabetics, pregnant or lactating women, the elderly and the poor. The consumption of empty calories, like processed food and restaurant food, is another risk factor for malnutrition. The problem is even worse when more than one of these factors is present.

Most of the time, nutrient deficiencies are only marginal, causing no significant signs or symptoms and giving no evidence of organic disease. Yet, these deficiencies adversely affect the body's ability to maintain health in the face of biological and psychological stressors. Numerous biological changes are now known to be associated with marginal deficiencies. These include increased susceptibility to infection, the promotion of degenerative tissue changes, and the slower healing of injured or degenerated tissues.

With aging, the need for certain nutrients increases but, unfortunately, the ability to absorb these nutrients decreases. This phenomenon contributes to the susceptibility of the elderly to many chronic diseases. In fact, some of those chronic diseases happen to people in their mature age. Just ask around: many people you know have already been diagnosed with deficiencies of vitamin B, vitamin A, calcium, iron, omega-3s and others.

Deficiencies of important nutrients have an immediate and direct consequence on cartilage, musculoskeletal and neurological structures.

To sum it up, it is necessary to correct nutritional deficiencies for people living in the United States. There are two ways to do so – by nutrient repletion and nutrient therapy.

Nutrient repletion is accomplished by improving the diet. A varied diet, rich in nutrients and poor in "anti-nutrients," is the first step in correcting these deficiencies. This is the diet we call the Jupiter Institute Omega Diet described in Chapter 7, a diet that should keep people in the "omega-3/antioxidant" state (which I also call "omega-3/good-eicosanoids-antioxidant" state), instead of the "omega-6/free-radical" state (which I also call "omega-6/bad-eicosanoids-free-radicals" state).

Sometimes, however, an improved diet is not sufficient to result in adequate nutrition repletion. A patient may fail to follow the diet over the long term, perhaps because of lack of motivation, knowledge or means. When dietary recommendations are not adequate to correct the nutritional deficiencies, nutrient therapy is required.

Nutrient therapy means taking nutrient pills, often at dosages well in excess of the recommended dietary allowance, for the purpose of preventing or treating nutritional deficiencies. This is accomplished through the ingestion of vitamins, minerals and supplements, also known as micronutrients, in the form of tablets and capsules.

While thousands of articles support the use of micronutrients, most publications agree that liberal consumption without guidance is irresponsible and dangerous and may do more harm than good. Nutrient therapy is not a matter of taking a few vitamins because you read that they are good for you, but rather of seeking guidance to find which supplements are most needed.

I don't want you to get the idea that if you just take a particular vitamin that you will be fine. If you suffer from chronic pain, arthritis, injuries, neck and back pain or neuropathies, taking vitamins and supplements is NOT the solution, but part of a sound program.

So, please don't make the mistake of thinking that a handful of pills will fix your problem. That is the passive-pill-taker attitude that rarely works in the eradication of pain conditions. Instead, assume the active attitude of incorporating the various therapies and lifestyle changes we encourage.

Our program combines seven approaches: medical care, diet adjustment, physical therapy, exercise, acupuncture, chiropractic care and nutritional supplementation. Taking supplements without considering the other treatments may not yield any improvement; the use of nutritional supplements is just one of several simultaneous therapies that you will need to follow. An updated list of recommended books on vitamins and supplements can be found at our website (www.jupiterinstitute.com).

VITAMINS

The vitamins with the greatest therapeutic effect for arthritis are the ones with active antioxidant properties: vitamin A, vitamin C, vitamin E and some of the B-vitamins.

Vitamins B1, B6 and B12 play an important role in the functioning of the nerves and are important additives in the treatment of painful neuropathies. Additionally, vitamin B12 nourishes bone marrow, which prevents anemia. Overall, B-vitamins are known to relieve headaches: vitamin B6, in particular, is known to fight pain. Supplementing the diet with B-vitamins is recommended for anyone who is struggling with pain and injuries. It is usually recommended to take supplements containing all the B-vitamins (B-complex) since they are more effective when the entire complex is taken together.

The combination of B-complex with vitamin A, vitamin C and vitamin E is the core of most nutritional supplement programs. However, excessive amounts of B-complex or dubious brands may cause adverse reactions. The same is true of poor quality B-vitamins.

Vitamin C and vitamin E have powerful antioxidant and anti-inflammatory effects, but they must be taken in correct amounts to be effective. It is unwise to overdo a good thing. Vitamin C helps in tissue repair and injury healing. Vitamin E protects tissues against damage caused by free radicals and improves nerve function. Vitamin E is also known to protect omega-3 fatty acids against free radical attacks.

Cautions

Because high levels of vitamin A can be toxic, it is safer to take mixed carotenes, which convert into vitamin A in the body. B-vitamins, mainly B3 (Niacin), B5 (pantothenic acid) and vitamin B6 (pyridoxine) play a role in the maintenance of multiple tissues, but excessive intake can cause adverse reactions.

Vitamin D and folic acid are two vitamins that, although essential for the structure of tissues, cause adverse reactions when taken in excess.

The problem when buying vitamins is that although there are hundreds of brands, most products do not contain what the label says. Many brands of vitamin C have no vitamin C at all in the tablet. Many bottles of vitamin B and vitamin E contain only a fraction of what the label says. Unaware of this, a person may take four or five vitamin tablets a day, but their minimal nutritional content provides no benefits. Some dubious brands may even have impurities that can cause immuno-allergic reactions.

We encourage readers to consult with their doctors or a local health food store in order to learn about high-quality supplement products. We also invite you to check the "Vitamins and Supplements" section of our website (www.jupiterinstitute.com) where we post some of the brands that we have found to be reliable. Saving a few dollars every month by buying cheap vitamins may adversely affect your health.

Also, don't be misled by marketing strategies that lead you to take supplements you don't need and at doses you should avoid: read, gather information, talk to your doctor, and learn before you put an unknown chemical in your body.

Excessive vitamins

Taking excessive amounts of vitamins can be risky and counterproductive. Doing this for just a few days may not cause a problem. However, when an individual who suffers from an ailment, or who is debilitated by age and inflammatory or degenerative conditions, takes excessive amounts of vitamins (especially those of poor quality), unpredictable adverse effects can occur. The old saying "the more the better" does not go for vitamins. Mega-doses of vitamins or supplements can be dangerous.

If you start taking a new vitamin or supplement and develop new symptoms, discontinue it and consult with your physician. However, some adverse effects like liver and kidney damage may give no symptoms; this is why we encourage you to keep in touch with your doctor when you start a new vitamin program, even if you feel well. Again, we invite you to consult our website, where we recommend several books on vitamins and supplements, or talk with the manager of the local health-food store. In general, people associated with local independent health-food stores are better educated on health and supplementation. Be as sure as you can that the manager is more concerned about health than in making a few extra bucks.

CARTILAGE-BUILDING SUPPLEMENTS

Glucosamine

Glucosamine is a supplement that provides raw material to rebuild damaged cartilage. Glucosamine is not as fast acting as NSAIDs; it is actually rather slow. Instead of just eliminating the symptoms, it works by healing the injured tissues that are the root cause of those symptoms. It also decreases the activity of the enzymes that attack the cartilage, helping to restore the eroded cartilage. People taking glucosamine decrease the loss of cartilage in the joints and on many occasions even gain new cartilage.

Glucosamine eases osteoarthritis pain by normalizing cartilage metabolism and promoting its healing. The most recommended type of glucosamine is glucosamine sulfate. Glucosamine chloride, another variety, is much less effective and should only be used by those individuals with an allergy to sulfur.

Many books and publications support glucosamine as an effective medication for arthritis, pain and inflammation. As mentioned above, the beneficial effects of glucosamine are slow to appear but long in duration. It takes 6-8 weeks before the benefits of glucosamine can be felt.

While those taking NSAIDs such as Ibuprofen and Naprosyn see the drugs' effect disappear after one to three days, those who have been taking glucosamine for any period of time find its effect lasting from 100 to 120 days after the glucosamine has been interrupted.

Caution: most glucosamine preparations are unreliable and may even contain impurities, so only certain brands are recommended. Many of the brands found in grocery stores and pharmacies do not contain what the labels say, or they contain the wrong type of glucosamine. Some brands bought by mail from unreliable sources are also of poor quality.

One study shows that 80% of the store brands are unreliable. Consumers of glucosamine, vitamins and supplements should be aware of misleading marketing strategies that may cause them to purchase a poor-quality product. We recommend that people avoid cheap store brands or fancy marketing labels. It is acceptable to save on paper towels and laundry detergent, but it is not safe to save on a product that is taken by mouth every day. It is not smart to buy cheap glucosamine, and other supplements. Again, please consult your doctor, chiropractor or local health food store for high-quality products.

Chondroitin

Chondroitin is a glycan compound required for the formation of cartilage proteins. It seems to protect joints from breaking down and its activity helps injured cartilage. It inhibits the action of destructive enzymes in the joint. Many publications describe chondroitin as a cartilage protector that works by stimulating the production of healthy cartilage, and by inhibiting the adverse action of eicosanoids. In all, chondroitin decreases inflammation and promotes cartilage repair in the arthritic joint. The recommended dose is 600 mg twice a day or 400 mg three times a day.

Some publications assert that chondroitin is not absorbed in the digestive tract, it is useless to take it, and that only injections of chondroitin are effective in decreasing pain and inflammation. However, whether it can be proven – or not – that the supplements are absorbed, we have seen chondroitin relieve arthritic symptoms time and again. Like glucosamine, many brands of chondroitin are not reliable and may even contain impurities, so consult a professional before purchasing.

Glucosamine and chondroitin combined

Many books and publications claim that the combination of glucosamine with chondroitin provides great success in the treatment of pain and osteoarthritis. Some authors, such as Dr. Jason Theodosakis, affirm that together they can halt, reverse and even cure arthritis. What is important about glucosamine and chondroitin together is that, unlike NSAIDs, they do promote healing of the damaged joint, albeit quite slowly. They alter joint structure favorably and interfere with the progression of disease. Numerous clinical trials have evaluated this combination and have demonstrated these benefits.

Overall, the combination of glucosamine and chondroitin has a positive structural effect in the joints that makes it very effective in the treatment of osteoarthritis and joint pain.

Similar to glucosamine, much of the chondroitin and the combined glucosamine/chondroitin products sold on the market today present the same challenges with purity, integrity and effectiveness.

This lack of consistency is so alarming that the *Journal of Rheumatology* evaluated these products with regard to quality, purity and concentration of ingredients. The result of this study showed that only 8% of the glucosamine and chondroitin products provide what the label says while more than 90% are unreliable. The unreliable brands not only provide products with lower quality and potency, but they most likely contain impurities that may cause adverse reactions. Only a handful of the over 200 brands of glucosamine and chondroitin are acceptable.

We recommend that you first check the label to make sure the product says "Made in the USA" or "Manufactured by XXX, U. S. A." Then, as mentioned before, consult a reliable professional – your physician, chiropractor or local health-food store manager – for guidance. You can also visit our website for guidance regarding vitamins and supplements.

SAM-e

SAM-e (S-Adenosyl methionine) is a sulfur compound used by the body to regenerate cells and reduce pain and osteoarthritis. It also decreases inflammation, and has a role in many chemical reactions in the body. SAM-e is often recommended for treating inflammation, arthritis and other painful conditions. It is believed to improve joint mobility. Clinical studies show that SAM-e relieves osteoarthritis, is well tolerated and is a promising therapy for relief from pain and swelling. The usual dose is 300-400 mg three or four times a day.

MSM

MSM (methylsulfonylmethane) is naturally produced in the body, but levels decrease with age and degenerative illnesses. Some publications assert that products with MSM decrease inflammation, relieve pain and spasm, and improve cellular function at the site of injury. The sulfur in MSM is thought to work as a kind of biological "cement" to help repair damaged tissue.

Other publications deny these statements saying that MSM has shown no clear benefits. These publications state that there are no human studies to show that MSM is effective in joint repair.

Our position in this argument is that it may provide benefits to many. Only recognized brands, however, are recommended. The recommended dose is usually 1,000-1,500 mg a day in divided doses.

MINERALS

Boron

Boron is a mineral that helps in the metabolism of calcium and magnesium and is important for bone health. It improves osteoarthritis and painful joints and has direct anti-inflammatory action. The recommended dose is 2-3 mg a day. Caution: it may raise estrogen levels.

Copper

Copper is an essential mineral, important in the synthesis of fibers for the support of the tissues. Excessive intake of zinc and iron may cause copper deficiency. The recommended dose is 1-3 mg a day.

Selenium

An essential mineral and a powerful antioxidant, selenium is often deficient in people with inflammatory conditions. Selenium fights free radicals and protects cells. Proper intake is recommended, but excessive intake could cause toxicity. Selenium also binds with mercury (ingested when eating contaminated fish) and blocks its toxicity.

Zinc

Zinc is essential to many body functions and its deficiency may result in joint pain.

Magnesium, Iron, Manganese and Copper

These minerals work together to help control joint metabolism, activating enzymes and promoting an anti-inflammatory effect. They ease pain by affecting the causes that trigger it.

Iron

Disease can result from either excessively low or excessively high intakes of iron. Some people do need to take iron supplements with their vitamins, but we don't recommend it unless it is needed. There is plenty of iron in green leafy vegetables.

Iodine

Deficiencies of iodine can lead to degenerative illness, including muscle weakness and arthritis.

ENZYMES

Bromelain

Bromelain is an enzyme found in pineapple that has been widely used to treat athletic injuries. Studies have shown that bromelain has anti-inflammatory properties. It helps break down the fibers that accumulate in the inflamed area. Bromelain apparently also decreases the formation of damaging inflammatory eicosanoids and promotes the action of the good anti-inflammatory eicosanoids. Caution: It may enhance the effect of blood thinning drugs, and may cause excessive bleeding in the case of a cut or injury for people taking these medications. The recommended dose is 400-1,000 mg a day.

HERBS

Boswellia serratia

This is a botanical product that has been used for centuries to treat arthritic conditions, and it is known to have anti-rheumatic properties. It inhibits the bad eicosanoids produced by the white blood cells (called leukotrienes), thereby favoring the action of the anti-inflammatory good eicosanoids.

ANTIOXIDANTS

The unstable substances known as free radicals are harmful to the tissues of our body. Many publications confirm that excessive amounts of free radicals damage healthy cells through their potent, oxidative effect.

Antioxidants, found in fresh, raw foods and vegetables neutralize this harmful oxidative effect. Although a well-balanced diet provides a variety of antioxidants, it will likely fail to provide enough of a daily supply. Hence, it is necessary to supplement our dietary intake of antioxidants. Antioxidant supplements are vitamin A, vitamin B, vitamin C, vitamin E, selenium, copper, manganese, zinc, green tea, bioflavonoids, garlic, bilberry, astragalus and alpha lipoic acid.

Alpha lipoic acid improves insulin function, decreases blood sugar and helps metabolic function. It improves cell energy, cell repair and has a protective effect on vitamin C and vitamin E. It is helpful in many injury conditions and is an ideal supplement for people suffering from diabetic neuropathy.

OMEGA FATTY ACIDS

The healing role played by omega-3, omega-6 and omega-9 fatty acids in injury, arthritis, and pain is well known and has been reviewed in previous chapters.

There are three main sources of omega-3s: the marine source (EPA and DHA), present in fish and fish oil gel caps; the seed and nut source (alphalinolenic acid), present in flaxseeds, flaxseed oil, walnuts, and pumpkin seeds; and plant sources, including algae and the omega-3 vegetables (see page 135).

Omega-6 comes from many sources. As explained in earlier chapters, omega-6 fatty acids are generally pro-inflammatory, and their intake needs to be restricted. However, gamma-linoleic acid (GLA) is an omega-6 that behaves like an omega-3, with anti-inflammatory properties. It is found in borage seed oil, blackcurrant oil and evening primrose oil. It is good for you and available in most health food stores. A couple of capsules a day are an excellent addition to the Jupiter Institute Omega Diet and help the body to remain in an anti-inflammatory state. Depending upon body conditions and needs, the usual recommended dose of GLA is of 1-3 grams a day.

Omega-9 (oleic acid), present in olive oil and olives, and in avocados and macadamias, also reduces symptoms of inflammation.

Combinations of the three types of omega fatty acids have strong anti-inflammatory and tissue repair effects.

All omega fatty acids are best when taken straight from nature. The amount of omega-3 on the dinner plate is sometimes difficult to establish because of variations in the EPA and DHA content of different kinds of fish. Also, since preparation methods affect omega content, there may be no way to tell whether the person is getting enough or too little of the good omegas.

Therefore, we encourage our patients and readers to supplement their diet with gel caps of fish oil or salmon oil. It is an easy way to assure that the daily requirement will be satisfied, and to avoid the worry about how much fish we are going to eat daily. Besides, these gel caps are very practical, and easy to swallow, and good brands give no aftertaste. Some people may experience slight intestinal side effects from these supplements; the most common are belching, flatulence and lose stools. However, these side effects occur in only about 5% of the population and can be diminished by switching to an alternative brand.

For people who do not like fish of any kind or who get an adverse effect from the fish-oil gel caps, the solution is to take flaxseed oil, walnuts and walnut oil. However, these oils must go through an enzymatic conversion in the body into EPA and DHA to become useful. Not every individual has the metabolic capability to perform this conversion. Sometimes, this can be determined by evaluating HDL levels in the blood. These individuals, consequently, will not enjoy the health benefits of these fatty acids.

Therefore, we advise using ground flaxseed, flaxseed oil – plain or gel-cap – walnut oil and certain nuts as a complement rather than the primary source of EPA and DHA. It is our opinion that fish oil and salmon oil are still the best sources of omega-3 fatty acids for the human body.

Whichever is taken, the usual minimum amount is one or two gel caps a day. However, this depends on the situation. If a person is dealing with an acute inflammatory process due to an injury, or is experiencing advanced degenerative joint disease, the quantity needs to be increased to 5, 10, 15 and even more capsules a day.

Here are the conversions if taken by tablespoon. One tablespoon equals 3 teaspoons, and each teaspoon equals 4-5 gel caps. Therefore, one tablespoon of flaxseed oil or salmon oil is more or less the equivalent of 12-15 gel caps.

The addition of GLA is needed in inflammatory processes: it is found in borage seed oil, blackcurrant seed oil and evening primrose oil, with borage seed oil being the best of them. The dosage used in inflammatory conditions (arthritis, etc.) is in the range of 1.2-2.8 gm a day. You need to check the label and calculate the amount of GLA in each capsule to find out the number of capsules to take. Since different brands vary in the amount of GLA per gel cap, intake may vary from 5 to 25 capsules a day. We suggest you start with 1.2 gm a day (you need to check the amount of GLA in each capsule) and then increase according to the tolerance, instructions and your condition.

We recommend 100-200 IU of vitamin E and 500-1,000 mg of vitamin C to be taken together to protect the omega-3 from free radicals.

Flaxseed oil should be stored in dark containers or in dark capsules. When buying liquid flaxseed oil, buy it in dark containers that are sealed airtight. Buy small bottles because it spoils easily. Smell it before you use it: it is okay if it smells like nuts, but it is not okay if it smells like paint.

Only certain brands of the salmon and fish-oil gel-caps are recommended. Consult your physician, chiropractor or health food store professionals to determine the brands of gel-caps of omega-3 oils that are recommended. You can check our website (www.jupiterinstitute.com), where we post some suggested brands.

WHICH SUPPLEMENTS SHOULD I TAKE – AND HOW MUCH?

Although the recommended daily allowances for vitamins and minerals are fairly small, for people facing pain, injury and arthritis these quantities are not adequate; supplementation is needed. However, the need for supplements and vitamins will vary depending on the problem the person is facing.

Different conditions require different types and quantities. Since the person will be taking these products on a daily basis, and for quite some time, it is important to understand what is being taken and why. Libraries and bookstores, where more detailed knowledge can be obtained, are excellent sources of information about vitamins and supplements, and of their applications and dosages. It does not take long and requires only a note pad and pen. As you review these books, you may be overwhelmed by the number of conditions and diseases that are mentioned. Focus on your condition and look for its treatment. Repeat the process with other books, and look for a general consensus about the treatment. If all books agree that Product A is good for your condition, you have discovered something useful. Consulting with a physician, chiropractor or a local health food store professional is also advised. You can also consult our website (www. jupiterinstitute.com) about recommended products and books to complement and enhance your knowledge of supplements.

Our recommendations regarding vitamins and supplements are not rigid but adapted to the individual. The requirement, tolerability, and amount of the supplement may be affected by a person's height, weight, allergies and sensitivities, current medication program, or other medical problems. It is most important that all these factors be taken into account, which is why we encourage consulting local professionals.

What follows are our general recommendations. Again, they need to be adapted to each individual. Pregnant women, people with debilitation, and those taking prescription medications must avoid taking anything unless it is approved by their doctor.

Again, we emphasize that supplementation is only one part of our seven-point program. The reader may not like or may not be able to follow all six of the other treatments we also recommend, but at least three are a must for proper repair and relief of inflammatory conditions.

The quantity of supplements to take and the length of treatment will depend on improvement of symptoms, durability, adverse reactions and the opinion of your physician.

Dosages also vary according to the quality of the person's nutrition. People whose diet consists of mainly meat, dairy and fried food, without raw vegetables, raw fruits, or fish require a larger and more frequent dosage of supplements. Those who follow a dietary program such as the Jupiter Institute Omega Diet need far fewer supplements. Certain conditions may demand a greater intake of particular supplements, even if the person follows a proper diet. Accordingly, the dosages we describe here should be used as a guideline only. Discuss specifics with a physician, nutritionist or a reliable manager of a health-food store.

Let me give you some examples. A one-and-a-half-pack-a-day smoker who eats very few salads and fruits needs a lot more antioxidant supplementation than a non-smoking vegetarian. A middle-age woman who follows our recommended diet of vegetables, fish, grains, olive oil, nuts and fruits, needs a lot less omega and vitamin supplementation than a woman whose main diet is packaged snacks, beer, junk food, pasta, pastries, sugary drinks and fried food.

General recommended doses

Calcium – 1,000-2,000 mg a day
Chondroitin – 300-400 mg 3 times a day OR 400-600 mg twice a day
Folic acid – 200-1,000 mcg (micrograms) a day
Glucosamine sulfate – 500 mg 3 times a day OR 750 mg twice a day
Manganese – 1-2 mg a day MSM – 500 mg 3 times a day
Selenium – 25-100 mcg a day
Vitamin A – 3,000-10,000 IU a day, or natural beta carotene 5,000-10,000 IU/day (IU=International Unit)
Vitamin B1 (thiamine) – 5-10 mg a day

Vitamin B12 (cyanocobalamin) – 25-50 mcg a day
Vitamin B2 (Riboflavin) – 5-8 mg a day
Vitamin B3 (Niacin) – 25-100 mg a day
Vitamin B5 (pantothenic Acid) – 25-50 mg a day
Vitamin B6 (pyridoxine) – 1020 mg a day
Vitamin C – 250-2,000 mg a day – some individuals may benefit
    from an even larger dose
Vitamin D – 200-400 IU a day
Vitamin E – 100-400 IU a day
Zinc – 15-50 mg a day

In the following sections, recommendations for particular conditions are given.

Injuries

In cases of muscular injury, ligament and tendon lesions, or injuries to any extremity, it is advisable to supplement the medical treatment with fish or salmon oils to provide omega-3 fatty acids. Taking antioxidants every day is also recommended, but the amount of each depends on the magnitude of the injury and inflammation. Three to 15 and even 20 capsules of salmon oil may be required every day in doses divided appropriately for the individual. Treatment is short – two or three weeks. Our Jupiter Institute Omega Diet is a must.

Neuropathies And Pinched Nerves

Individuals struggling with these conditions need the addition of a B-complex. Depending on the case, one-half a tablet a day up to one tablet twice a day (of the B-50 preparation) may be needed, but the duration of treatment is determined by your physician. Check to see if you have any allergies before you take any product. It is a good idea to complement the B-complex with antioxidants. You may take B5 once or twice a day. If you are struggling with an active bulging disc, with pain in your arm, shoulder or leg (sciatica), you can take one B5, one antioxidant, and three to five salmon oil gel-caps while your primary doctor coordinates the rest of the treatment.

The addition of fish or salmon oil depends on the cause of the neuropathy and the situation of the spine. It is necessary to evaluate how much degeneration, deviation and inflammation are present.

Arthritis

In the case of osteoarthritis and chronic joint disease, glucosamine and chondroitin are strongly recommended. The standard dose of glucosamine sulfate is 500 mg and chondroitin 400 mg, each taken three times a day.

Fish or salmon oil should be taken as well according to how much of the joint is degenerated and whether there is more inflammation or degeneration present. Doses of 3 to 12 gel-caps a day divided into two or three doses should be sufficient. People who are allergic to fish oils should take flaxseed oil instead. The dosage of this oil should start at 3 gel caps a day and then increase according to the patient's condition. Some authors recommend giving 2 capsules and then 3, later 4 and 5 capsules, three times a day. Some recommend even more, reaching as many as 25 capsules a day. Remember, this is an equivalent of about 1½ to 2 tablespoons of liquid oil, and it depends on how inflamed the joints are.

In severe cases of neuropathies or arthritis, you can use liquid fish oil (or liquid salmon oil), a good tablespoon twice a day, with meals, for several weeks. The conversion is 4 - 5 gel capsules equal one teaspoon, and 3 teaspoons equal a tablespoon.

A daily antioxidant is recommended to protect the omega-3s and to block free radicals. Some individuals may also benefit from taking GLA (borage seed oil or evening primrose oil) for its anti-inflammatory properties. A good starting treatment can be: a glucosamine/chondroitin capsule, one borage seed oil capsule, one antioxidant, and two salmon oil gel-caps three times a day. Later on, double the salmon oil.

Results will not come quickly; it takes time for all these compounds to work at the molecular level. It is acceptable to take NSAIDs during this waiting period since they not only relieve the symptoms but also decrease inflammation and allow the supplements to work.

Tendonitis, Bursitis and Inflamed Ligaments

When these conditions are of recent onset, they have a strong inflammatory component at their core. Accordingly, in addition to medical treatment, we recommend the addition of fish or salmon oil, antioxidants and GLA in the form of borage seed, blackcurrant or evening primrose oil. Protocols depend on how much inflammation is present. A recommended starting plan is one complete antioxidant per day, four to six salmon oil gel-caps per day, and GLA twice a day, increasing as advised. You should see a physician, chiropractor, or a physical therapist to get a proper diagnosis, keeping in mind that on occasions a cortisone shot can help significantly with these conditions. (You can get this from a rheumatologist or orthopedist.)

Sizeable Areas of Inflammation

Significant inflammatory conditions such as severe arthritis, inflamed muscles and tendons, muscular injuries, acute sprains and bursitis may benefit from the following combinations:

Omega-3 oil (fish, salmon or flaxseed oil):
- For people up to 125 pounds – 4-8 gel caps a day
- For people 125-150 pounds – 8-14 gel caps a day
- For people 150-200 pounds – 14-20 gel caps a day

    (If you prefer liquid form: 1 teaspoon= 5 gel caps; 1 tablespoon= 3 teaspoons=15 gel caps)

Multivitamin/antioxidant complex containing: (if possible, all in one tablet)
- Copper & Zinc – trace
- Folic Acid – 0.5-1 g
- Selenium – 5-25 mg
- Vitamin A – 10,000 Units of B-Carotene
- Vitamin B1 (thiamine) – 5-6 mg
- Vitamin B2 (riboflavin) – 5-7 gm
- Vitamin B3 (niacin) – 40-80 mg
- Vitamin B5 (pantothenic acid) – 6-8 mg
- Vitamin B12 (cyanocobalamin) – 25-50 mcg
- Vitamin C – 500-2,000 mg
- Vitamin E – 50-250 IU

Also:

- Gamma-linoleic acid (GLA): minimum 240-320 mg a day, up to 1.2-2.8 grams a day
- Omega-9 (olive oil): 2 tablespoons twice a day
- Consider also adding low doses of boron, MSM (methylsulfonyl-methane) and copper.

Neck Pain, Back Pain And Chronic Osteoarthritis

These conditions require omega-3 fatty acids and antioxidants, but the dose depends on the severity of the condition and how advanced it is – especially how much inflammation is present. The more recent and active the condition, the more antioxidants and omega-3s needed to fight inflammation. In addition to the other therapies mentioned, start with low doses of GLA, omega-3s, omega-9s and antioxidants, and slowly increase the dosage. A good combination is one GLA, one B-50, three omega-3s, and one antioxidant, twice a day. Our Jupiter Institute Omega Diet is a must, along with a visit to a doctor since you may need X-rays, chiropractic manipulation, physical therapy, acupuncture, or a cervical collar or special pillow.

Other supplements for arthritis include bromelain, zinc, copper, boron and MSM, all of which have anti-inflammatory properties that may help with inflammatory conditions. The dose for MSM is 1,000-1,500 mg a day, which may cause diarrhea. In this case, cut back to one-half of the recommended dosage. Bromelain can be given at 400-500 mg, three times a day. The dose for boron is 1-2 grams a day. Since human beings are all different, some may find better relief with bromelain and MSM than with glucosamine/chondroitin.

Again, if you have any of the conditions mentioned here, it is useless to just take pills if you aren't also adjusting your diet as we outline in the chapter on the Mediterranean Diet, and you aren't participating in three or more of the other therapies we describe in this book. Vitamins or supplements are NOT the solution; they are only part of the program. Consultation with a physician is a must.

THE CRITICAL IMPORTANCE OF CHOOSING RELIABLE BRANDS

Unreliable products, purchased out of convenience or for their cheap price, may not only be ineffective but may cause adverse reactions and even allergies. Companies dedicated to providing high-quality brands regularly test their products using national protocols. They also employ manufacturing techniques that avoid the use of contaminates and solvents, and control the quality of the ingredients. Only a few companies provide products of good quality. Remember you are taking these products every day for the purposes of healing, so you need to use a good product.

As with cars and furniture, cheap brands give you unreliable products. The general public needs to be aware that many of the manufacturers of glucosamine, chondroitin, vitamins and minerals are based in foreign countries, which may not have governmental agencies such as the U.S. Food and Drug Administration that vouch for the safety and efficacy of products of this kind.

Many of the foreign suppliers not only provide poor quality supplements, they have problems with the hygiene of their workers and the plant. Since they are untouchable by American authorities they succeed in supplying our market with inferior and sometimes unsafe products. Some authors suggest that 80-90% of the supplements sold in pharmacies, grocery stores and even health food stores should be avoided.

We recommend, again, to check with your physician, chiropractor, other medical professionals, or the manager at your local health food store to determine the best brands.

Just a few weeks ago I convinced a man with heart fibrillation to stop taking those "high quality" vitamins he was getting by mail from some wonderfully marketed website. Ten days later his heart stopped fibrillating. I also see people with indigestion, irritable bowel, liver disorders, skin troubles, etc, all due to the adverse effect and cross-reaction of the multiple vitamin pills they take. Some of those reactions are likely due to the interactions of probable contaminants and impurities.

POINTS TO REMEMBER

Remember, taking vitamins and supplements could be useless if:

✦   that is all you do to improve your condition and you don't care about the other six points of our program: diet change, medical care, physical therapy, chiropractic treatment, acupuncture and exercise.

✦   you take cheap, unreliable brands that give you uncertain amounts of the active ingredient. Buy supplements from reliable sources that clearly state "Made in U.S.A.", and don't be swayed by fancy marketing.

✦   you take incorrect amounts. If you under dose, you are missing out on the nutritional benefit that is needed to heal your condition; if you overdose, you run the risk of toxicity.

✦   the pills are outdated. Check the expiration date.

✦   you are taking the wrong nutrients for your condition. An example of this is taking lots of B-complex and vitamin C for degenerative knee disease, but not also taking glucosamine.

CHAPTER TEN

Body and Mind Exercises for Recovery

 The benefits of exercise are great, but the potential for injuries and harm caused by exercise is also great. In other words, exercise can help you but it can hurt you as well. What to do?

Well, here's what not to do: don't let the fear of injury stop you from exercising. Choosing not to exercise will work against you. Although professional guidance is recommended in most instances, only minimal instruction is needed when embarking on an exercise regimen.

A regular exercise program is beneficial for anyone who suffers from any form of an arthritic condition.

Over the last decade, many studies have shown that exercise reduces joint pain and stiffness while increasing muscle strength and flexibility. According to the Arthritis Foundation, study after study confirms that those who exercise are healthier, live longer, and cope better with pain and injuries from arthritis.

- In one important study, a group of people were placed in a supervised exercise program that included exercises for flexibility and strengthening as well as aerobic exercise. MRI imaging was used to measure the thickness of their knee cartilage before the exercise program began and several weeks later. The new MRI images showed that exercise had increased the thickness of the cartilage – a significant beneficial change since thicker cartilage improves the physiology of the joint.

• In a study conducted at Wake Forest University, about 300 elderly people with osteoarthritis of the knee were divided into three groups. Each group was confined to only one type of therapy. The first group got only health education, the second group performed aerobic walking exercises, and the third group did strength training. After 18 months, those who received health education remained in the same condition as before, while the two active groups reported feeling better, having less pain and stiffness and better joint function.

• A similar study at Tufts University's Center for Physical Activity and Nutrition recruited 46 people with crippling arthritis, who experienced pain and stiffness every day. This study was unique in that a therapist visited patients in their homes, and instructed and trained them on exercises consisting mainly of stretching and flexibility combined with strength-training exercises. Half the participants did this active exercise, but the other half – the control group – received mainly a short lecture and emotional support. No specialized equipment or tools were used.

After four months, the difference between the two groups was remarkable. Patients in the exercise group had considerably less pain, and their physical function had improved significantly. They were able to walk, go outside, get in and out of their cars, sit, stand and even climb stairs with greater ease. They slept better, and there was a noticeable improvement in overall quality of life. Those who did not exercise and received only emotional support and health education – "someone to listen to them" – showed very little improvement.

The conclusion that we can draw from these studies is clear: you must exercise in order to improve an arthritic condition.

REST AND YOUR ARTHRITIS WILL GET WORSE;
EXERCISE AND YOUR ARTHRITIS
WILL GET BETTER

ACT!

As you peruse this chapter, it is important for you to understand that simply reading it will not bring improvement. I say this because I have seen obese people attending lectures on weight loss and then taking no further action. I know people who go to financial conferences and do nothing with the advice they receive. I have met heart patients on diuretics who sit through a two-hour "seminar and bagels" conference. They listen and say "Oh, that is very interesting," or "Oh, he's such a good speaker," but they do nothing to change their habits.

In general, people seem to think, "I went to the lecture and that is enough." Or, they say, "Hey, I am trying." But the only effort they have made is to attend the lecture: when they get home they do nothing with what they have learned.

If this is your attitude, please go no further. No amount of reading is going to do you any good. However, if you are reading with the intention of changing and improving, this book is an extremely valuable tool. There are other books we recommend: *Strong Women and Men Who Beat Arthritis* by Miriam Nelson, Ph.D. (G. P. Putnam's Sons, New York), *Reverse Arthritis & Pain Naturally: A Proven Approach to an Anti-inflammatory, Pain-free Life* by Gary Null, Ph.D. (Essential Publishing, North Palm Beach), The Arthritis Foundation's *Guide to Good Living with Osteoarthritis,* and several other books mentioned on my website (www.jupiterinstitute.com).

To get better, there are two things that you need:

1. You need to understand the process of arthritis, injuries and inflammation, which I have described earlier in this book. The better you understand it, the better you can address it.

2. You need to assume an active attitude and lifestyle in which you acknowledge that you have full responsibility for your own care. You need to tell yourself "I want to get better, and in order to get better I need to make some changes." If not you, then who? And if not now, then when?

BENEFITS

The benefits of exercise are documented in many books and publications. Patients with osteoarthritis, back pain and injuries credit exercise programs with reducing their pain and improving their function. Most authors encourage individuals with chronic pain (regardless of cause) to do some type of exercise and stretching on a regular basis. For people with pain, stiffness, and stress, exercise provides a beneficial combination of healing and relaxation that contributes to the repair process.

Regular exercise decreases the pain and limitations of arthritis and may also reverse a bit of the joint degradation. It is now recognized that some of the symptoms associated with arthritis may, in fact, be due to inactivity.

Exercise benefits the entire organism by:

- improving strength and flexibility;
- decreasing stiffness and pain;
- improving balance and muscle endurance;
- improving the cardiovascular and pulmonary systems;
- promoting relaxation and stress reduction;
- improving insulin sensitivity, sexual function, sleep and even resistance to disease;

- improving blood pressure and managing hypertension;
- assisting in controlling weight and reversing obesity;
- improving mental alertness and sleep patterns.

Beyond these general benefits, exercise helps the joints by:
- improving joint biomechanics;
- stimulating the flow of joint fluids;
- strengthening the muscles, tendons and ligaments around joints;
- keeping joints healthy and functional;
- improving blood flow to the areas affected by arthritis and inflammation.

To many doctors and patients, exercise seems to be counter productive for an arthritic joint. When a joint is swollen, tender, or stiff, it seems that exercise will make it worse. But, as mentioned earlier, many studies have shown this assumption to be false. Moreover, there are plenty of testimonials from my patients for the tremendous benefit of exercise in the arthritic joint.

IT IS NOW RECOGNIZED THAT SOME OF THE SYMPTOMS ASSOCIATED WITH ARTHRITIS MAY ACTUALLY BE DUE TO LACK OF EXERCISE

Of course, appropriate rest helps reduce joint inflammation. But it is also an established fact that excessive rest decreases the functional capacity of the limb and is deleterious to health. Too much rest reduces fitness: muscle tissue wastes away or turns to fat, tendons and ligaments weaken and contract, joint cartilage degenerates. Given this, it is paradoxical for physicians to recommend rest for chronic arthritis and painful conditions.

With an appropriate exercise program, arthritic patients can safely improve their strength and enhance their functional capacity. Increasing the strength in the muscle improves the performance of many everyday activities and relieves physical and psychological discomfort.

HELPING YOUR MUSCLES

As we discuss the multiple benefits of exercise, we also need to consider the effect on muscular tissue. Exercise increases muscle activity, demanding a greater supply of oxygen, glucose, nutrients, minerals and vitamins. Proper nutrition is essential to satisfy your muscles' requirements for water, protein and natural carbohydrates. Recommended foods are lean meats and low-fat cheeses, fresh vegetables, nuts, calcium-enriched rice and soy milk, whole grains, fish and green leafy vegetables.

For those who engage in vigorous exercise or significant sweating, we recommend replenishing potassium with fruits, pumpkin seeds, potatoes (preferably sweet potatoes and always with the skin), and bananas. For people who exercise on a regular basis, we also recommend the intake of supplements. It is difficult to follow a diet that will provide all of the vitamins and minerals that a muscle needs without supplementation. Vitamin B could easily become depleted, as could vitamin C and other vitamins. Taking vitamins will nourish the muscles and protect them against possible damage during exercise.

Additionally, antioxidants protect muscle tissue against the damaging effect of free radicals. Vitamin C, a well-known antioxidant, reduces swelling and repairs tissue. Omega-3 fatty acids reduce the inflammation of the muscle and promote tissue healing. A multivitamin tablet supplies a host of vitamins required for the healing of ligaments and tendons. Glucosamine provides the raw material required by the body to regenerate ligaments and tendons and repair cartilage, which are all strained during intense activity.

If you have read the earlier sections in which I talk about supplements, you know that I consider choosing high-quality brands of supplements to be of utmost importance. I explain why in Chapter 9, where the main discussion of supplements is found.

FINDING THE RIGHT TYPE OF EXERCISE FOR YOU

I encourage all patients in the Jupiter Institute Pain Program to exercise regularly. For anyone who is suffering from pain, arthritis and injury, however, I say: choose your exercise wisely. No matter how good an exercise can be in many situations, it can further damage a joint, ligament or tendon that is already hurting.

The improper type of exercise can increase irritation of a bursa, and cause a worsening of bursitis. The wrong type of stretching may further strain or sprain a ligament or muscle that is already damaged. A bad disc or swollen cartilage may get worse with inappropriate exercise. If you are obese, jogging or walking five miles may aggravate hip and back conditions, and if you have a whiplash injury you can actually make things worse by going to the gym.

The solution to all of these potential problems is to participate in the correct type of exercise with proper frequency and intensity. But how does an untrained person know what exercise is best, and how often and how intensely they should practice it? Should you consult your doctor? Many physicians, internists and family doctors know little about the subject and, unfortunately, try to guess. Should you look in a book? Books can provide so many options that you may end up feeling overwhelmed and have no sense of what to do.

The solution is to ask the two types of professionals who know best about exercise: chiropractors and physical therapists. Don't ask anyone else! Few other professionals know so much about neuromuscular anatomy, joint physiology, body mechanics, human biophysics and healing techniques.

Sooner or later you will likely visit (or at least consider visiting) a chiropractor or physical therapist to receive care for your pain, arthritis or injury. Use this wonderful opportunity to ask what type of exercise is best for you and what type to avoid. Also ask how intensely, how often, and for what length of time you should engage in a particular type of exercise, as well as the best combination of stretching, aerobic and strength-training exercises. Ask again and again, and take notes.

Ideally, it is best to integrate your exercise with a treatment plan designed by a physical therapist and/or a chiropractor. Your exercise should be part of this treatment plan, and you should follow the recommendations of those who are treating you.

Of course, it is important to find a good chiropractor and physical therapist. Ask your doctor, friends, relatives or neighbors. Don't allow yourself to be guided by fancy marketing. Seek, visit and inquire. Being well informed may actually determine whether or not you recover.

ALL PAINS ARE NOT THE SAME!

I talk about different types of exercises in the next section: flexibility exercises, strengthening exercises, aerobic exercises, even sports. However, I don't want to go too deeply into the subject for three reasons. First, it is not the main goal of this book. Second, I would need a whole book, with pictures, to teach you exercises and how to do them. Third, I think that exercises need to be taught one-on-one by a therapist or a qualified trainer. Yes, you can use books as a guide, but an individual program for you – including what kinds of exercise to choose, how many different exercises, when to exercise and for how long, what exercises not to do and when not to exercise – needs to be taught in person by someone who knows this field very, very well.

For example, take shoulders: a stiff, tender right shoulder is not the same in a 78-year-old woman who stays at home as it is in a 55-year-old man who works in a supermarket and plays tennis. These two individuals, both with similar complaints of pain and stiffness, need to be evaluated by a physician and then sent to physical therapy (and perhaps to a chiropractor as well) for evaluation, treatment and exercise instruction. One of them may have torn ligaments and tendonitis; the other may have a partial tear in a muscle with significant cartilage degeneration. The symptoms – pain and stiffness – may be similar, but the problem is different and requires a different approach.

In the case of the knee, imagine three individuals: Bobby, a surgeon who plays soccer on weekends; Jeannie, a busy landscaper; and Martin, 60, who used to play basketball twice a week until six years ago when he became a businessman. Now he does not participate in any physical activity. All three come to my office with the same complaint: pain, stiffness and mild swelling in the left knee. Well, the knee may look the same in the three of them. Should the treatment and exercise be the same? Let's take a look.

Bobby's knee is strong and without degeneration, but he has a partial tear in the medial ligament and bursitis next to the patella. Jeannie's ligament and tendon are fine, but she has degeneration in the cartilage with inflammation and spurs. Martin, on the other hand, has a partially torn meniscus along with tendonitis. The treatment for these three patients should not be the same. The exercise prescribed should not be the same either.

As much as I enjoy exercise books, I maintain that there is nothing better than the personal guidance of a therapist. Although I read books and know a lot about exercise, when I injure myself I seek guidance on recovery and exercise instruction from qualified professionals. In these two cases: fishing a shark in Islamorada, which lead to a frozen right shoulder, and pulling a tree from my backyard (which my wife had warned me not to do), which resulted in a torn hamstring ("Serves you right!" she said), I turned to the combined treatment efforts of physical therapist and a chiropractor. They pulled me through and helped me get better faster.

Types Of Exercises

Although there are multiple types of exercises, we can reasonably divide them into four groups: *Flexibility, Strengthening, Aerobics* and *Sports.*

Flexibility exercises move the joints and muscles through their full range of motion, gradually increasing how far they can move and the ease with which they move. As the joints become more mobile, they are able to function more effectively with less pain. These exercises help relieve stiffness, and when done correctly, have beneficial effects on inflamed joints, tendons and ligaments.

Flexibility exercises mainly involve stretching to decrease stress, help heal lesions in the muscles, improve posture, and provide relief. However, over-stretching or stretching with improper motion may cause muscle and ligament injury. Have your therapist instruct you in the proper technique.

Strengthening exercises increase the power of the muscles that move, protect and support the joints. They counteract the muscular wasting and weakness that often accompany painful joints. Strengthening exercises improve muscle mass and muscle function, which directly and indirectly improve the physiological function of the joint. Blood flow to the tissues is improved, providing oxygen and glucose and eliminating waste products. This is extremely beneficial for the healing of injuries, arthritis and areas of inflammation.

Strengthening exercises dramatically improve joint function and decrease pain. Light weights are often used in this phase and are very helpful. Have your therapist instruct you on the type of strengthening exercises that are best for your condition.

Aerobic exercises enhance overall fitness by stimulating the lungs and the cardiovascular system. They improve the body's energy balance by energizing joints, muscles and tissues overall. The term aerobic, when applied to exercise, means that the person is able to breathe normally while doing this activity. This is a moderate type of exercise in which you will be breathing deeper and fuller but without the panting and rapid breathing of fast ("anaerobic" exercise). During aerobic exercises, the heart and lungs work harder, you breathe a bit harder, and your heart rate is increased.

Sports activities can be done alone or in groups. They increase muscular activity and make the heart and lungs work a lot harder. This may be beneficial in many situations, but it can be counterproductive. Group sports activities (basketball, soccer, swimming teams, etc.) are not recommended because they may push people to exercise much more than what is permissible for arthritic joints, injuries or areas of inflammation. Solitary sports activities (swimming, jogging, etc.) may provide important benefits so long as certain parameters are observed. These parameters should be established by a health professional (a physician, a chiropractor, or a physical therapist) since they depend on the type and location of the injury, the number of injuries or affected joints, the weight of the person, and the type of sport activity.

ADDITIONAL INFORMATION

We have found the following books to be excellent sources of information about exercise:

The Arthritis Foundation's Guide to Good Living with Osteoarthritis – a publication of the Arthritis Foundation.

Arthritis: Your Complete Exercise Guide, by Neil Gordon, M.D.

Exercise Beats Arthritis, by Valerie Sayce and Ian Frazer.

We also list a number of other useful books on our website, all of which can be found in your local library or bookstore.

As an arthritis, pain, or injury sufferer, you should integrate exercise with physical therapy or chiropractic therapy, excellent anti-inflammatory nutrition (the Jupiter Institute Omega Diet), adequate sleep, perhaps a short course of medication (your medical treatment), and specific supplements. It is also advisable to consider acupuncture, if indicated.

PRECAUTIONS AND GUIDELINES

Here are some points to bear in mind prior to and during exercise:

1. Make sure you do not have any **medical conditions** that may worsen with inappropriate exercise. Talk to your doctor; a medical evaluation may be needed. Do not exercise if your doctor tells you that you have active cardiopulmonary disease, infectious or febrile illness, or severe vascular disorder.

2. **Start slowly.** Do not perform exercises either too intensively or too frequently in the first few weeks of the program.

3. Choose forms of exercise that **minimize the stress** to painful, inflamed or damaged joints or muscles.

4. **Know when to stop.** Don't push yourself beyond your limits. If a movement hurts, stop and evaluate what has happened. Pain is a warning that you are causing damage to your body. The old cliché "no pain, no gain" is a dangerous misconception.

5. **Don't overdo it!** You are here for the long run, and you don't want to abuse your body.

6. **Don't exercise if your joints are severely inflamed.** When joints, muscles and tendons are hurt, swollen and very tender, exercise could actually worsen the condition. Consult with your doctor or therapist if this occurs.

7. Never exercise to **show off.**

8. **Choose exercises and activities that appeal to you**. Do not do any exercise just because it is popular.

9. **Competitive exercises are not good for arthritis.** They add extra strain to tissues and joints. Attempting to perform as well as others may end up pushing your muscles, ligaments, joints and tendons to levels of function for which they are not prepared.

10. **Respect gravity.** If you suffer from low back pain, hip trouble or even a knee disorder, jogging and long-distance walking may cause more harm; if you are obese the effects are generally worse.

11. **No alcohol or meals** before exercise.

12. Do not exercise near **bedtime,** or the energizing effect may keep you awake.

13. **Stretching:** don't do it unless you know how to do it properly. Don't improvise. Ask your therapist how and when to stretch, or you may end up hurting your ligaments, tendons and muscles.

14. **Warming up** is an important phase of exercise – see the heading below. If you are unsure how to warm up, ask your therapist.

15. **Swimming and water activities** are excellent for people with arthritis, inflammation and injuries.

16. **Going to a gym** may or may not be a good idea. On one hand, gyms give you tools for good exercise, such as exercise mattresses, weights, machines, stationary bikes, rowing machines and so on. On the other hand, they are often full of people who are showing off, and their presence could make you feel uncomfortable or out of place. If you would like to join a gym, choose one where you are comfortable.

17. **Don't skip your exercise** just because you're short on time. Even if you have only 10 or 15 minutes to exercise, go ahead. Doing something is far better than doing nothing.

18. **Try to exercise all parts of your body.** You can achieve this by combining the treadmill with floor exercises or the stationary bike with some weights. Some parks offer exercise stations where you combine exercises of different parts of your body. Don't forget your abdominal and back exercises.

19. **I advise against push-ups.** They cause excessive strain on joints and muscles; don't do them, as they may hurt you.

Warming Up

It is a good idea to warm up your body before you start exercising. Arthritic joints and injured muscles or tendons can stiffen very easily, particularly if you have not done any exercise for a while. Warming up is a gentle way of starting to move, and it helps to get joints and muscles ready for exercise.

Once muscles start working, blood flow increases and tissues become better prepared for exercise. You should not do stretching at this stage, because stretching cold tissues may cause micro-tears and other damage.

The warming-up phase can be started either sitting or standing. Then, completing a full repetition of each, do a series of the following: raise arms over shoulders, flex (tighten the muscles) the arms, raise shoulders without raising the arms, gently clap the hands forward, raise one knee then the other, rotate the body to the right and then to the left, slowly bend forward and then slightly backwards, perform a mid-level squat. On the floor, sit up and, bracing your knees, roll down slowly onto your back; raise one leg 45 degrees, and then the other. Do all these exercises in very slow motion, causing minimal stretching. You can also do a slow military march, moving your arms in circles while doing front circles or side circles. Again, do all these very slowly, while taking slow, deep inhales while forcing the air out of your lungs completely on the exhale.

TAI CHI AND YOGA

Tai chi and yoga represent a class of exercise that differs from the classic "stretching-flexibility-strengthening" programs currently employed by conventional medicine. They bring many benefits and are highly recommended for the appropriate patient. Both yoga and tai chi originated in South Asia; they are highly successful complementary therapies with centuries of knowledge and proficiency behind them. Both incorporate a mind-body approach to the rehabilitation of disorders like pain, injury, arthritis and multiple neuromuscular disorders. They are also extremely effective for reducing stress.

Yoga and tai chi include movement in slow motion, body positions, meditation and breathing techniques – but they are far more than that. When done properly, they have an effect on the energy of the body and mind. Indeed, yoga and tai chi are like icebergs: they are a lot deeper than they appear.

To enjoy the benefits of yoga and tai chi, you must understand them and accept their principles. As a first step, you need to accept a difficult concept to visualize and comprehend: Your bio-electricity is not like a battery driving your heart, but rather like a flow of vital forces that run through your body like a river. Many people are oblivious to it, but it is there, flowing like water through your limbs, skin and organs. Tai chi and yoga, in their different ways, exert an influence on this flow of energy, providing strong and highly favorable effects. They offer additional benefits to each of the Jupiter Institute Pain Program therapies that we describe in this book. Both require careful instruction.

Tai chi

Tai chi is a gentle exercise program that is part of traditional Chinese medicine. Derived from the martial arts, tai chi is composed of slow, coordinated movement, meditation and deep breathing, which help correct imbalances in joints, nerves and muscles and enhance physical and psycho-emotional health. Practicing it encourages positive biological and psychological effects for people of all ages.

Many studies, journals, and books state that tai chi improves neuromuscular function, lessens the pain of arthritis and fibromyalgia, and enhances flexibility and strength. Tai chi is, in addition, an excellent complementary therapy for a wide range of conditions, including gout, heart disease, hypertension, headaches, sleep disorders, anxiety, depression, stress and even asthma.

History. The principles of tai chi were born from a blending of Chinese martial arts with the philosophical idea of Taoism. This was a combination of two antagonistic ideas: the sophistication of martial arts, which attempts to overpower and hurt the enemy, and the Taoist principles of gentleness and yielding. This synthesis was originated some eight centuries ago by a Taoist priest who used his fundamental wisdom of self-defense and philosophy to create the soft, slow movement of a non-combative martial art.

This ancient form of movement is still a daily routine for millions of people across China. It was introduced to the United States in the early 1970s and has since grown in popularity.

The idea behind this wonderful exercise is that the energy of the human body, Qi, flows in the body through many channels. When Qi flows properly, the body, mind and spirit are in balance and health is maintained. The slow movements of tai chi facilitate the flow of this essential bio-energy through the body. Tai chi movements emphasize the importance of weight transference, which is an essential component of good balance. Through gentle and fluid movement, it improves posture, coordination and gait.

Tai chi has three major components:

Movement: slow, gentle movement, full of grace and coordination that looks like both a dance and a slow-motion Chinese martial arts fight.

Meditation: practitioners meditate (acute mental focus) as they exercise. This soothes the mind, enhances concentration and reduces anxiety. Tai chi is a "meditation-in-motion" exercise.

Deep breathing: deep inhalation and exhalation provide fresh oxygen to tissue and brain while improving lung capacity and blood circulation.

Tai chi is an exercise that anyone who can walk can perform safely, taking the joints gently through the range of motion, stretching muscles and tendons while emphasizing deep breathing and meditation. Classes are inexpensive and tai chi can be practiced almost anywhere at any time, with no special equipment or clothing. The beneficial effects of tai chi make this unique meditation-in-motion exercise a great addition to any pain or arthritis management program.

Tai chi improves overall fitness, coordination and agility. People who practice it on a regular basis tend to have good posture, flexibility and coordination. They are more mentally alert, sleep better at night and suffer less pain.

Tai chi is endorsed by the Arthritis Foundation for the treatment of pain and arthritis. A study at Case Western Reserve University in Cleveland, Ohio showed that tai chi reduces the intensity of arthritis pain and has a strong beneficial effect on chronic joint pain.

Tai chi improves balance, thereby decreasing the risk of falls; it also provides improved postural stability while decreasing neck and back pain.

In March 2004, the *Archives of Internal Medicine* reported that tai chi provides physiological and psychosocial benefits and is a safe and effective way of promoting balance control, flexibility and coordination.

In September 2003, the *Journal of Rheumatology* reported that tai chi improves the pain, swelling and stiffness of arthritis, improving physical function and quality of life for people with osteoarthritis.

Certainly, tai chi is a great addition to the therapy we describe in our Jupiter Institute Pain Program. It complements the therapies and enhances their beneficial effects.

Tai chi can be practiced in addition to your favorite exercise, and can be done before or after your routine. It is also an excellent addition to the exercises taught to you by your physical therapist and your chiropractor.

Learning tai chi. Don't try to learn tai chi from a video or book. Learn it from a teacher who can make sure that you are doing the movements correctly. Choose your teacher carefully. Tell your instructor about your aches, pains, injuries and arthritis. Be realistic: tai chi is not a treatment but rather a complementary therapy for pain, arthritis and injury.

Yoga

Yoga is neither a religion nor just a series of postures. It is a philosophy of life and a powerful system of self-awareness that uses low-impact activity. The motions and positions that are so typical of yoga represent just a portion of this otherwise very complex mind-body program.

Yoga's capacity to increase good health and well-being is well documented, with numerous books and journals attesting to its medical benefits. For many people, yoga has proven to be a safe and effective way to alleviate many forms of neck and back pain.

Yoga can provide several healing benefits for people with various types of strain. It can also help in the healing of injured muscles and in decreasing the time of recovery from an injury. Studies have shown that yoga may provide a treatment option for patients with osteoarthritis by decreasing pain and disability. More than 75 trials have been published about yoga in major medical journals. These studies have shown that yoga is a safe and effective way to increase physical activity, increase muscular strength, improve flexibility and promote relaxation. It increases body energy and decreases aches and pains.

Yoga is a meditative form of exercise that stretches and strengthens muscles, increases range of motion, improves circulation, empowers the natural power of the human body and significantly enhances the quality of life. There are many styles of yoga – from gentle to athletic – practiced today. Beginners should always stick with gentle styles of yoga.

Yoga teaches the basic concept of mind-body unity: if the body is sick and suffering, mental health will be affected, and if the mind is stressed and agitated, the health of the body will be compromised. Hence, the integrated healing of mind and body is the main goal in the practice of yoga.

Background. Yoga originated in India some 5,000 years ago, which makes it perhaps the oldest mind-body health program known to man. It combines philosophical ideas, spiritual concepts about bio-energy, and physical exercises that were taken from observation, experience and immense knowledge. Yoga was developed as a way to access, build and nurture our natural energies. It was created also as a philosophical compilation of techniques, positions and motions that provide spiritual advancement and a practical way of self-improvement. Various schools of yoga emphasize different techniques, but they all teach a methodical practice of breathing, meditation, contemplation, physical postures, mental concentration and a path to awaken spiritual awareness.

Practice. Many hospitals across our nation provide yoga classes for multiple purposes. Cedars Sinai Medical Center in Los Angeles encourages yoga as a way to improve cardiovascular disease, decrease blood pressure and improve blood sugar control. They use yoga for their cardiac rehabilitation patients.

Stress reduction and relief from fatigue are two of the many benefits of yoga. Some centers offer yoga as a way to improve fertility; others offer it for people suffering from pain or recovering from injury. Researchers at the UCLA Medical Center in Los Angeles found that just four weeks of regular yoga sessions significantly reduced the frequency and severity of chronic pain.

Today's yoga participants are young and old, flexible and stiff, slim and overweight, men and women. They are everyday people who are just like you but who want to treat their bodies well and cure their ailments without pills, doctors or side effects. Yoga is especially good for people with arthritis and pain because these conditions tend to reduce confidence and self-esteem while yoga increases them.

Multiple publications have reported that yoga improves strength and flexibility, decreases stress and anxiety, and is an excellent tool for pain management. A study at the Western Virginia School of Medicine analyzed the effect of yoga therapy for lower back pain and found that patients practicing yoga experience a reduction in pain intensity and functional disability and they use less pain medication.

Some of the beneficial clinical effects of yoga include:

- **Cardiovascular:** decreased heartbeat and blood pressure
- **Musculoskeletal:** increased strength, flexibility and range of motion of joints, and improved balance
- **Joints:** relief for stiff, damaged and arthritic joints
- **Mind and Nervous System:** enhanced alertness, memory, concentration and focus, less fatigue and stress, greater relaxation and lower emotional tension
- **Lungs:** more efficient breathing and blood oxygenation
- **Digestion:** better digestion and less constipation
- **Pain:** reduction in pain and improvement in painful conditions through beneficial stimulation of the pain center (the part of the brain responsible for sending messages to areas of the body)

A word of warning. Although practicing yoga brings many benefits, the number of injuries caused by this exercise is increasing. Doctors and physiotherapists are reporting an upsurge in the number of inexperienced students injuring themselves after straining to get into difficult positions. This may be due to improperly trained instructors and over-motivated, eager-to-perform students. Yoga injuries are mainly caused by strain and over-stretching of ligaments, tendons, nerves and muscles. It is recommended to join only yoga centers in which the instructors are fully trained, certified and proficient; learning from poorly trained instructors at sports centers is strongly discouraged. Find a qualified instructor, and avoid pushing your body too fast or too hard to reach positions that you are not accustomed to. Progressing slowly while releasing the need to compete are both extremely important in yoga.

CHAPTER ELEVEN

"Mediterraneanizing" Your Diet

This chapter aims to show you another way of following the Jupiter Institute Omega Diet, so you can improve your overall health. Being in the omega-3/antioxidant state will also help you fight your pain, arthritis or injury more successfully. In Chapter 7, we discussed which foods are good to eat and which are not. Now you will learn that some foods usually considered "bad" or "not OK" can be converted ("Mediterraneanized") to make them healthier. Yes, you may be able to go back to steak and pasta by following some simple rules.

The countries that surround the Mediterranean Sea have a rich tradition of fine food, a tradition that has been spreading throughout the world. Mediterranean cuisine has achieved international popularity not only because of its fine flavors and aromas but because it is recognized as being the healthiest in the world, in tune with modern trends in nutrition and health.

Fifteen countries and three continents border the Mediterranean Sea: to the north, the European countries of Spain, France, Italy, Greece and Turkey. To the east is the Asian continent with Lebanon, Israel and Syria. To the south is the African continent with Morocco, Egypt, Libya, Tunisia and Algeria, and the island nations of Cyprus and Malta. Each of them is unique in their language, culture, tradition and also in cuisines, spices and food presentation.

Despite these differences in culture and cuisine, many ingredients, spices and recipes are common to the entire region. Indeed, when perusing books on Middle Eastern, French, Spanish, Italian and Moroccan cuisine, it is fascinating to see how some dishes have traveled around the region. Slightly modified, seasoned with local ingredients, given different names, they become typical dishes of many different areas.

Among the staple ingredients of Mediterranean cuisine are couscous, rice, vegetables, spices, olives, fish and olive oil used copiously.

Of all the Mediterranean countries, Greece is the country whose diet has been shown to offer the best health benefits. Accordingly, we are going to take the Greek cuisine as the model Mediterranean Diet.

Although dishes from other Mediterranean countries will be considered as well, dishes that deviate too much from the typical Greek style, or offer foods that are too far removed from the omega-3 stream, are not recommended even though they are considered Mediterranean dishes.

This is the concept that differentiates the Jupiter Institute Omega Diet from the Mediterranean Diet: certain dishes, although they are Mediterranean and generally considered part of the Mediterranean Diet and Mediterranean culture, are so loaded with omega-6s and carbohydrates that we discourage their consumption. Examples are the pasta with meatballs and fried tomato sauce of Italy, the pork dishes of Spain, the cochinillo of Segovia, the falafel with hummus of Israel, and the tahini and pita of Lebanon and Egypt. The same goes for kebabs, kibbeh, fancy risottos, etc., and for many fried dishes and desserts, including fried calamari, baklava, fried cheese, etc. Several typical Greek dishes are left out for this same reason: they deviate from the omega-3 stream.

Caution: you can find many "Mediterranean Diet" books out there with wonderful dishes and enticingly beautiful photographs of foods. However, the fact that a dish is in such a book, or that a dish is labeled Mediterranean, does not make it good for you.

Don't be misled! When choosing a Mediterranean dish in the books commonly found in libraries, bookstores and even on our website (www.jupiterinstitute.com) you must keep in mind the classifications we provided in the Nutrition chapter. We classify the foods that provide omega-3s and antioxidants, and the ones that flood the body with omega-6s.

"MEDITERRANEANIZING" YOURSELF

As you plan or prepare your food, remember the important principles of the Mediterranean Diet: the low level of omega-6s, the high level of antioxidants, and the abundance of omega-3s and omega-9s. As you learn about different Mediterranean dishes, you will analyze each recipe and adjust it to what we teach you here. Some dishes, such as fried dishes or pork dishes, you will not be able to use. Others, however, you can adjust, for example by replacing fried snapper with grilled cod. Hence, you will "Mediterraneanize" the dishes to subtract omega-6s and add omega-3s and omega-9s (olive oil). You can even buy a Mediterranean Diet cooking book and write adjustments for each recipe. Where it says fry, write bake, poach or grill; where it says pork, scratch it out; where it says chickpeas or green peas, decrease their amount and add beans; and where it says pasta, substitute rice. Increase the olive oil in each recipe. In short, "Mediterraneanize" the Mediterranean dishes – or maybe we should say "Omeganize" them.

As you go through this process we want to remind you of the reason why antioxidants are important: they protect your omega-3 essential fatty acids. If this is not taken into account, you may find yourself with a dish that contains a good amount of omega-3s but no antioxidants. Then a good chunk of the omega-3s you've consumed may end up being destroyed by omega-6s and free radicals. Therefore, it is important to consume the omega-3s accompanied by its "bodyguards," the antioxidants.

You will find antioxidants in the following foods:

- fresh raw vegetables
- fresh herbs (basil, chives, cilantro, dill, garlic, ginger, parsley, rosemary, thyme)
- fresh raw fruits
- red wine

You will find the good omega-3s and omega-9s in:

- oily fish (salmon, sardines, tuna, herring, cod, mackerel, blue fish, trout, anchovies)
- nuts (walnuts, macadamias, hazelnuts, almonds)
- avocado
- olives, olive oil
- omega-3 vegetables (spinach, arugula, lettuce, kale, collard greens, alfalfa sprouts, broccoli, watercress, cauliflower, bean sprouts)

How can you "Mediterraneanize" a steak if it's all omega-6? Make sure it's grilled, not fried, and eat it with olive oil and a spinach and broccoli salad.

How can you "Mediterraneanize" pasta? Eat it with olive oil and some of the good fish mentioned above. Or, mix it with a sauce made from olive oil, walnuts, fresh basil and a bit of parmesan cheese.

How can you "Mediterraneanize" fish? Have it poached, baked or grilled, then once on the plate, drizzle with olive oil and eat it with fresh, raw vegetables.

How can you "Mediterraneanize" pork or fried chicken with corn? You can't. Just forget them – "Mediterraneanization" has its limits! Hot dog, hamburger or pizza? Sorry.

And here we offer some interesting news. For the same reasons, we exclude some high omega-6 Mediterranean dishes, many non-Mediterranean dishes from countries in other parts of the world can be "Mediterraneanized" to suit our program. There are ways to prepare Mexican dishes and Chinese dishes in a Mediterranean way. Japanese, Brazilian and even New Orleans favorites can be adapted to the Mediterranean-Greek style and suddenly become transformed into healthy dishes. You can read a cookbook and "convert" – "Mediterraneanize" – some of the recipes to make them acceptable.

Let me give you an example: pasta with fried tomato sauce and meatballs is clearly out of bounds. But if you chop fresh garlic, fresh basil and some olives, mix them with olive oil and pour the mix over plain pasta, then you'll have "Mediterraneanized" pasta and yes, you can eat it.

As a general rule, we recommend staying away from fried oils of any kind. But it is okay on occasion. Lightly steam some chopped vegetables, then mix them with brown rice and very slightly sauté them with olive oil, soy sauce, Mirin and garlic powder for "fried rice à la Mediterranean." Don't laugh! It's healthier than the standard version.

You need to learn to make your dishes omega-friendly, which means to decrease the omega-6s and increase antioxidants, omega-3s and omega-9s. Fried catfish with a glass of beer is not the same as poached salmon with a drizzle of olive oil and a glass of red wine.

As you explore all of these concepts, remember that food from restaurants, cafeterias, take-outs and fast food restaurants, as a rule, are not Mediterranean; they are unsafe in terms of dieting, and generally unhealthy.

JUPITER INSTITUTE OMEGA DIET RECIPES

Chapter 7 gave you the theory behind our Jupiter Institute Omega Diet, now for some practical tips. My aim here is not to write a cookbook, but to show you some dishes that give you an idea of how easy it is to follow Mediterranean guidelines. I invite you to think about food differently from this point forward.

"Mediterraneanize" or "omeganize" your meals because that is what creates a healthy body. You can also describe it as making your food "Omega friendly."

Before we move on to recipes, let's recapitulate the essential points: the Jupiter Institute Omega Diet is low in omega-6s and rich in omega-3s, omega-9s (olive oil) and antioxidants. It is based on the classic Mediterranean Diet, yes, and is very similar to it.

But this is how our diet is different:

A. It tells you, upfront, which foods are good for you and which are not, clearly establishing these guidelines from the beginning.

B. It modifies ("omeganizes") many Mediterranean dishes. It forbids and thus eliminates other Mediterranean dishes (because they are deep-fried, and have excessive carbohydrate content and, therefore, an unfavorable omega balance). It allows many non-Mediterranean dishes as long as they are "Mediterraneanized." We make you aware of these principles so that you know what you are doing.

With the Jupiter Institute Omega Diet, you know what you are eating and become aware of the omega-3, omega-6, omega-9 and antioxidant content of every meal.

This is not a cookbook, but the following recipes can be used as a guide to help you make nutritional decisions.

SPREADS

Bruschetta Romana
Coarsely chop and mix:
2-3 medium tomatoes
2 green onions
2 sun-dried tomatoes
4 black olives
Fresh basil
2 tablespoons olive oil

Mix and add salt, ground pepper and add a bit of grated Parmesan cheese. Spread over toast or bread.

Tapenade (Olive Spread)
Finely chop and mix well:
¾ tablespoon lemon juice
1 teaspoon Dijon mustard
4 black olives, 4 green olives
½ cup olive oil
4 tablespoons capers
Pinch of ground pepper
½ can anchovies
1 teaspoon white wine or brandy
1 garlic clove, minced

Mix well and spread over bread, toast or hard boiled eggs.

Love your bread?

You just love bread and don't want to give it up? Then "omeganize" it. Every time you eat bread, dip it in olive oil. You can prepare a quick sauce with olive oil and some herbs or spices and then soak the bread in this mix. Or use fish oil or flaxseed oil. And have some walnuts with it. By doing this you are enriching your body with omega-3s and counteracting the adverse effect of the flour.

Pasta Sauces

Fine Herbs Pasta Sauce

Mix well:
½ cup olive oil
Salt

Your favorite combinations of dry herbs such as rosemary, marjoram, oregano, thyme, etc.

Let stand for 10-15 minutes before serving.

Sicilian Sauce For Pasta

Finely chop:
1 onion and 2 garlic cloves

Sauté with olive oil Spray on a Teflon pan. Then remove from heat and place in microwave dish and add:

¼ cup olive oil
1 or 2 teaspoons capers
2 tablespoons canned tomato paste
4 teaspoons cracked pine nuts
2 teaspoons chopped black olives
Salt

Mix well and heat in microwave. (You can heat it in a frying pan also, as long as you sauté just a few minutes and not at maximum heat). You may add more tomato paste if you like. Serve over pasta.

Fine Seasoning Pasta Sauce

Mix well:
½ cup olive oil
Salt

Add your favorite seasonings in the preferred combinations such as curry, ground cumin, ground bay leaves, thyme, chili powder, turmeric, onion powder, paprika, etc.

Add 1 tablespoon store-bought pasta sauce and mix well.

Puttanesca Pasta Sauce

In small skillet sauté with olive oil spray:
1 medium onion, minced
3 garlic cloves, minced (do not allow garlic to burn)

Then add:
2 tablespoons chopped sun-dried tomatoes
1 can (14 oz.) crushed tomatoes
Ground black pepper
Salt
1-2 pinches of red pepper
1-2 pinches of white pepper
2 teaspoons olive oil
You may add more red and white pepper if you wish.

Lightly and briefly sauté this mix and add:
1 (2 oz.) can anchovies
6 chopped black olives
1 teaspoon fresh oregano
1 tablespoon balsamic vinegar

*Lightly sauté again (be very quick). Remove from heat and let cool.
Add ¾ cup of olive oil and mix well.*

Pesto Pasta Sauce

Mix well:
3 tablespoons finely chopped basil (fresh)
½ cup olive oil
2 cloves garlic (minced)
Salt

Add 2 teaspoons Parmesan cheese and ½-¼ cup chopped walnuts.

A word about pasta

Pasta is without a doubt delicious. However, it is also dangerous. We all know that pasta is fattening, but that's not the issue here. Pasta has an adverse effect on inflammation. It pushes the eicosanoid system to produce harmful inflammatory eicosanoids. The more pasta you eat, the worse the effect. Consequently, the only way to eat pasta and avoid this effect is to balance it strongly with omega-3s and omega-9s. Forget about eating pasta with meat sauce and meatballs – that is asking for trouble. Mix the pasta with olive oil (omega-9) and have it with salmon or tuna (omega-3) and some red wine.

You can flavor the olive oil with some store-bought pasta sauce. We give you some pasta sauces in this chapter, but you can find many more in a variety of cookbooks. Just remember to Mediterraneanize the sauce!

RICE

Spanish Chicken Paella

- Use a large skillet with cover.
- Chop and sauté with olive oil spray: 1 onion, 3 cloves garlic, then add 1 can of chicken broth (after skimming off the fat) and 1 can of water.
- Add a pinch of salt, freshly ground black pepper, 1 tablespoon of white wine, and between ¼ and ½ teaspoon of saffron or yellow coloring powder, which (you can find in the market's spice section).
- Mix and measure up to 1⅓ cup of chopped green and red bell peppers, green peas and green onions, and add them to pan.
- Add cubed, raw chicken, about ⅔ lb.
- Bring to a boil.
- Add 2 cups of uncooked rice: bring to a second boil, and then leave on low heat and cover. If you want to add other spices such as curry, thyme, oregano or ground bay leaves, do so before the second boil.
- In 18 minutes it is ready. Uncover, add olive oil generously (⅓-½ cup) and mix it well.
- For Mexican paella add, before the boil, a bit of corn, chopped onion, chili powder, and ground cumin, then, just before serving, a bit of chopped fresh cilantro.
- Notice that green peas and corn are used only in small amounts for garnishing.

Cuban Rice And Beans

- Prepare rice: Boil 3 cups of water with a pinch of salt and add ⅓ cup of plain beef broth.
- Add 1⅔ cups of uncooked white rice.
- Bring to a boil, lower the heat, cover and simmer for 18 minutes.
- Then remove from heat. Add 1 can of black beans or red beans (drained and washed well) and 4 tablespoons of olive oil. Add the spices and seasonings that you like (hot sauce, habanero sauce, curry sauce, Louisiana hot sauce, etc.)
- Mix thoroughly and serve.

Turkish Raisin Rice

Mix in a pot:
3 cups water
$\frac{1}{3}$ teaspoon salt
$\frac{1}{2}$ teaspoon yellow food coloring or turmeric
After mixing, bring to a boil and then add:
1$\frac{1}{2}$ cups of uncooked rice
2-3 tablespoons raisins
2 tablespoons pine nuts

Bring to boil again, cover and simmer for 18 minutes. Uncover and add 2-4 tablespoons of olive oil, mix well and serve.

Thai Rice

Place 2 tablespoons of grated coconut in dry pot. Place on stove over medium heat, move and fluff it with a fork. It will toast very quickly, so pay attention and remove from heat when almost done. It is extremely easy to burn this! Coconut should be slightly brownish but not dark.

When ready, add:
3 cups of water and bring to a boil
1$\frac{1}{2}$ cups uncooked rice
Salt
2 teaspoon minced ginger

Bring to a boil and then cover and simmer for 18 minutes. Add plenty of olive oil before serving. You can mix the olive oil with some curry and Tabasco sauce for enhanced flavor.

Easy Yellow Rice (make s 3 cups)

Mix in a bowl:
2 cups water
Salt
garlic powder
½ teaspoon of saffron or yellow coloring powder
½ cube chicken or vegetable bouillon

Bring to a boil and mix, then add 1 cup of uncooked white rice and boil for another 15-20 minutes. (Note: brown rice is healthier but takes longer to cook – approximately 45 minutes. Adjust recipe cooking times when using brown rice.)

Bring to a second boil, cover, and simmer for 18 minutes. Remove from heat, add olive oil, mix well and serve. You can enhance the flavor of the olive oil with a spice of your choice.

Chinese Fried Rice

In a large skillet sauté with olive oil spray:
¼ onion (minced)
3 cloves garlic (minced)

Remove from heat and let cool

Add:
3 cups cooked white rice
¾ tablespoon olive oil
Soy sauce (to taste)
Mirin cooking wine (to taste)
1 cup of your favorite vegetables (already steamed) such as peas, carrots, snap peas, green pepper, red pepper, celery.
1 teaspoon of fresh minced ginger

Optional: add 1 small can of drained bamboo shoots or water chestnuts. Place back on stove – mix as you heat, but don't cook – and serve promptly.

Jamaican Rice

Prepare as above, but add 1 teaspoon of curry powder after the first boil.

Cuban Rice With Chicken
Prepare as above, but before the water starts to boil, add:
2-3 cups of cubed raw chicken
A little more salt
Another pinch of garlic powder
1 tablespoon white wine
1 teaspoon of olive oil

After bringing to a boil, add the rice, bring to a second boil, let it simmer covered for 18 minutes.

Remove from heat, add at least 4 tablespoons (or more) of olive oil, mix well and serve.

SALADS, SALSAS, DRESSINGS AND MORE

Simple Salad
Mix chopped raw vegetables of your choice, using vegetables of at least three different colors! Add salt and a generous portion of olive oil. Commercial salad dressing, Parmesan cheese and croutons are all forbidden.

Mediterranean Herbal Salad
As above, with the addition of chopped, fresh herbs of choice (see list) and the addition of dry herbs of choice (see list), and plenty of olive oil.

Louisiana Collard Greens
(Cook this outside: collards have a powerful smell when cooking!)
Sauté 3-4 large handfuls of collard greens in olive oil, adding
1-2 beaten eggs
Salt
½-¾ chopped apple

It is ready when the eggs are scrambled.

Mexican Salad

- In a tray or deep dish, place a layer of chopped lettuce, followed by a layer of chopped multicolored vegetables including tomato and 2-4 tablespoons of corn.
- Then spread ½-1 teaspoon of ground cumin and chili powder and 2 tablespoons chopped cilantro, pour on olive oil – generously
- Salt to taste
- Spread irregularly with a layer of: 1-3 tablespoons of fat-free sour cream, 1 can of red beans, sprinkle 1-2 teaspoons lime juice, throw in 6-8 chopped black olives.

Mix as you serve.

Acropolis Salad

Mix 5 cups chopped raw vegetables of several colors (at least 3 different colors), then prepare the dressing:

½ cup walnut pieces

½ cup olive oil

2 tablespoon white wine

1 tablespoon lemon or lime juice

½ cup chopped olives (green or black)

2 teaspoons capers salt and pepper

Mix well and serve.

Mexican Pineapple Salsa

(To add to salads, chicken, fish or beans)

1-2 cups chopped, raw, ripe pineapple

Salt

1 tablespoon finely chopped fresh cilantro

½-1 teaspoon ground cumin

2-3 teaspoons lime juice pinch of black pepper

2-3 teaspoons of finely chopped onion olive oil (generously)

½-1 teaspoon Tabasco or your favorite hot sauce

Mix well and let stand before adding to your meal.

Couscous

Prepare the grain, following the instructions on the box; when finished and on the plate, add at least 2 tablespoons of olive oil.

Walnut Couscous

Add a pinch of grated Parmesan cheese and a large tablespoon of chopped walnuts to the water before adding the couscous.

Moroccan Couscous Salad

Finely chop:
2 tomatoes
1 bunch of green onions

Add:
¼ cup minced parsley
1 tablespoon minced fresh cilantro
½ cup olive oil
1 tablespoon lemon juice
Salt and pepper

Slightly mix and add 1½ cups of cooked couscous. Mix well. Serve.

Variations: Use chopped mint instead of parsley, adding chopped cucumber. Or replace the parsley and cilantro with 1 tablespoon of chopped, fresh rosemary and a pinch of marjoram.

Mediterranean Beans

1-15 oz. can red kidney beans
2-3 chopped tomatoes
A few thin slices of onion
1 tablespoon chopped basil
Salt and pepper
4 tablespoons olive oil
¼-½ tablespoon lemon juice

Mix well and serve. Replace the chopped basil with ½ tablespoon chopped fresh rosemary for a more Mediterranean flavor.

Dry Bean Salad
Same as the Mediterranean Beans, but instead of basil use choice of
a: Mix 2 teaspoons fresh rosemary with a pinch of marjoram or
b: Mix ½ teaspoon thyme and ½ teaspoon oregano.

Mediterranean Bean Salad
*Add the Mediterranean Beans to 3-6 cups chopped multicolor
vegetables, and then add additional salt and plenty of olive oil.*

Tomatoes Espanioles
*Cut large tomatoes in half, scooping their pulp into a mixing dish.
Mix:*
Tomato pulp
Chopped canned tuna
1-2 tablespoons olive oil salt to taste
1-2 teaspoon mayonnaise

Fill the tomato shells and serve immediately.

Greek Salad
Chop:
1 head of lettuce
2 tomatoes
⅓ cup red onion
⅔ cup cucumber
½ cup red bell pepper
½ cup green pepper

Mix and add:
1 tablespoon finely chopped fresh parsley
½ cup crumbled feta cheese
10-12 chopped olives (green or black)

Mix well and let stand. For dressing, mix well:
⅓ cup olive oil
1 minced clove of garlic
2 teaspoon of fresh lemon juice
1-2 pinches of fresh rosemary

Mix well. Pour the dressing onto the salad when serving.

Caribbean Mango-Bean Salad

Mix together:

2 cups chopped lettuce

2 tablespoon corn

1-15 oz. can red beans

½ cup olive oil chopped cilantro

⅓ teaspoon ground cumin

1-2 cup chopped mango

Salt

Lime juice

Optional:

2 tablespoon of salsa, or

2 tablespoon of chopped tomatoes & onion

Mix well and serve.

New Orleans Creole Salad

Mix well and let stand:

5 large, very ripe tomatoes, sliced, then cut each slice in half

¾ medium-sized onion, finely chopped

Dressing:

1 garlic clove, minced

1 teaspoon Worcestershire sauce

¼ cup tomato sauce

½ teaspoon Creole or other mustard

¼ cup red wine vinegar

1 teaspoon sugar

½ teaspoon freshly ground pepper

½ teaspoon salt

1 tablespoon minced basil

½-1 teaspoon Tabasco

1 cup olive oil

Mix all ingredients well and let stand. Add to salad just before serving.

DRESSINGS

French Dressing

½ teaspoon salt
2-3 tablespoons lemon juice
Pinch of black pepper
½ teaspoon mustard

Mix well and gradually add ¾ cup of olive oil while stirring gently.

Herbed French Dressing For Salads

Prepare French dressing as above, adding
¼ teaspoon mustard
¼ teaspoon salt
Pinch of black pepper
¾ teaspoon of each of the following fresh herbs: chopped basil, thyme and sweet marjoram

Mix well.

Blue Cheese Dressing

Mix ½ cup of the French dressing with:
2 tablespoons olive oil
2-4 tablespoons crumbled blue cheese

American Blue Cheese Dressing

Mix well:
3 tablespoons of olive oil
2 teaspoons of mayonnaise
Add 2-3 tablespoons crumbled blue cheese

Italian Dressing

Mix:
¼-½ cup white wine vinegar or lemon juice
2 minced or pressed cloves of garlic
½ teaspoon oregano
¼ teaspoon dried dill
⅓ cup olive oil
¼ teaspoon chopped basil
1-2 teaspoons ground walnuts

Refrigerate until serving.

Meats, Poultry and Fish

Steak and Hamburger

The best way to eat these omega-6 products is to balance them with foods high in omega-3s and omega-9s. Prepare a multicolor salad or any one of the salads we mentioned here. It is even better if you use the omega-3 vegetables that we mentioned in the Chapter 7, p. 117. Then add a couple of tablespoons of olive oil onto the steak or hamburger. This way you will be balancing the omega fatty acids.

Chicken Fricassee

Place 4-5 breasts of chicken in a stewing pot. Add:

3 cups water

2 sliced carrots

2 stalks celery

1 large onion, chopped

8-10 mushrooms

Salt

1 tablespoon white wine, 1 teaspoon olive oil.

Bring to boil, then lower the heat, cover and simmer for 1 hour. Remove chicken. Strain the stock. Mix the vegetables with ¼ teaspoon of paprika and ⅓ cup of olive oil.

Mix well to make a paste. Place the chicken over rice and pour the paste on top of the chicken.

New Orleans Remoulade Sauce

(for chicken and turkey)

Combine:

¼ cup mayonnaise

½ teaspoon anchovy paste

1 tablespoon drained chopped capers

½ cup olive oil

2 teaspoon French mustard

1 tablespoon drained finely chopped green olive

1 teaspoon finely chopped parsley chopped cucumber pickle

½ teaspoon chopped, fresh tarragon

Mix well and pour over chicken.

Fried Fish and Beer

Use the white fish cod or mackerel with omega-3 (snapper, grouper, mahi-mahi do not contain omega-3). Cut into pieces. Fry in Teflon pan with olive oil and olive oil spray (half-and-half), on medium, but not high, heat.

Prepare sauce:
4 tablespoons olive oil, mixed well with:
2-3 teaspoons of either mayonnaise or tartar sauce.

Set aside.

When fish is ready, serve on the plate. As you eat, dip the fish in the sauce. Oh yes... the beer. Forget the beer! Serve with red wine.

Niçoise Salad

2 tomatoes cut into cubes
1 cubed cucumber
1 cup Bibb lettuce
6 fillets of anchovies
12 black olives
1 cup romaine lettuce

Mix well. Add French dressing (see page 226) to serve.

Anchovy Dressing

Mix ½ cup of French dressing (see page 226) with:
2 tablespoons olive oil
1 tablespoon anchovy paste

Acapulco Dressing (for meat, chicken or fish)

Mix ½ cup French dressing (see page 226) with:
2 tablespoons olive oil
3 tablespoons chili sauce
1 teaspoon of Tabasco

Sushi And Sashimi

Sushi and sashimi are two of my favorite foods.

Mix the wasabi, soy sauce and ginger with 2 tablespoons olive oil. Mix well. Dip each piece of sushi and sashimi into this mixture and eat as much as you want.

Chicken, Turkey, Fish à la Mediterranean

Sprinkle chicken, turkey or fish with salt and garlic powder. Grill or bake. Once it is on the plate, add the following sauce.

In a cup mix:
3 tablespoons olive oil
Pinch of salt
½ teaspoon lemon juice
1-3 teaspoons of:
- any ONE of your favorite sauces or dressings: Worcestershire sauce, mustard, ketchup, mayonnaise, horseradish sauce, hot sauce, red sauce, Chinese or Thai sauce, cranberry sauce, cheese sauce, or
- your favorite combination of chopped, fresh or dry herbs.

Mix well and let stand. Then pour on your dish. Soak every piece in this mix as you eat. Finish all the sauce.

CHAPTER TWELVE

Weight Loss Plan

 If you are overweight and suffering from arthritis and injuries, losing weight will relieve your symptoms and help the body repair. The aim of this chapter is to provide you with a low-calorie diet that you can use as a guide or reference if you need to lose weight.

Losing weight is not a simple process; it is a rather complex metabolic one that is different for each individual. People react in their own way to different weight-loss diets, and the same weight-loss diet causes different metabolic reactions in each individual.

The 1200-calorie diet that we give you here is not the golden key, but rather a guide that you can use while being supervised by your primary care physician. Being overweight may be caused by overeating or a lack of exercise, but it may also have other causes. So, don't embark on a significant weight-loss program without first getting a check-up from your doctor, including EKG and blood tests.

Also, discuss this dietary plan with your physician before starting. You could have a metabolic problem such as diabetes, thyroid disease, hormonal imbalance or an endocrine disorder that may need to be investigated. Ask your doctor to review your medications, since certain medications are known to cause weight gain.

Bear in mind that this is a 1200-calorie diet. Depending on your constitution, you may need a 900-calorie per day diet or a 1500-calorie per day diet to begin. In these cases, the diet provided here may require adjustments. A similar nutritional protocol can be made for 800 calories a day, 1000 calories, 1500 calories and 1800 calories depending on the person's metabolism and the amount of weight loss needed.

This is not a regular low-calorie diet. It has been "Mediterraneanized." This plan is designed to give you restricted calories and to decrease omega-6s while increasing omega-3s, omega-9s and antioxidants. Accordingly, this diet will push you into a "favorable eicosanoid state," which I call the omega-3/antioxidant state. Some people may lose weight just by being in this state; we hope so! Whether you lose weight or not, this is a healthy, anti-inflammatory diet that will help your ligaments, tendons and joints.

Keep in mind that each person is different; some may need a high-protein low-carbohydrate diet, while others do better with less protein. Still, others may need more vegetables or a different schedule of meals. Additionally, this diet may need to be modified if the person suffers from a chronic condition such as diabetes or colitis. However, this is a well-balanced 1200-calorie diet that provides a good starting point: it balances proteins, fats and carbohydrates while providing an adequate amount of nutritional vitamins and minerals. The calculated grams of protein should satisfy the average person's need. The amount of essential fat has also been calculated – this plan provides an adequate amount of essential fatty acids in the form of omega-3s and omega-9s. Many dietary books have been consulted to develop this diet, and there is an abundance of valuable advice. This dietary program is also educational; it teaches you, for example, that you should never snack on just carbohydrates.

You will be following this program for several months if not indefinitely, since you need to learn how to disengage from the causes that led you to be overweight (habits, environment, carbohydrate abuse, snacking, emotional eating, restaurants, processed foods, societal stresses, etc.). Be clear about this: If you stop the program and re-engage in your previous practices, you will do so with a vengeance and probably regain all the weight you lost and more.

In this first phase, it is critical to adhere strictly to the plan, and eat only what the plan indicates and at the times the plan designates. As your work and activities expose you to other foods, snacks and treats, you must exercise control and stick to our program. Practice and you will acquire the automatic reflex of seeing other foods and saying to yourself "that's not for me."

If hunger, lack of satiety or cravings is a problem, don't cheat! Just call your doctor for advice. You must pre-plan your meals and daily activities ahead of time so you will have all the ingredients that you need for your meals. Exercise as planned; it is an essential part of the program. Exercise is especially helpful when you are feeling on the verge of spiraling out of control. Get out for a brisk walk with deep breathing; it can rebalance body chemistry and curb your appetite.

Ideally, this plan should be in effect for 6-8 months. During this time, it is best to go to your clinic or doctor's office one to two times a month for medical monitoring and counseling.

Diets can get boring after a while, so no matter how good this diet is, take time to research other diets and discuss them with your doctor. Also, talk to your doctor in advance about what to do when you fall into a rut. Most of all make sure you don't stop eating this way! If you do, you may gain back what you have lost. If you don't know what to do, or if you need some guidance, contact our office (mail, fax, e-mail, etc.) and we will help you with suggestions.

Remember: when you have a weight problem the problem does not disappear when you lose weight. Eating disorders have underlying emotional, mental and spiritual causes that need to be addressed simultaneously for successful long-term weight management. If you have abused food in the past, there is a predisposition to do so throughout life. Obesity in particular is a medical condition that can require lifelong medical supervision and treatment.

WHAT YOU CAN EAT

As you plan or prepare your food, keep these important principles of the Jupiter Institute Omega Diet (and the Mediterranean Diet on which it is based) in mind: the low level of omega-6 fatty acids in contrast to the important omega-3 and omega-9 content, as well as the high level of antioxidants.

You will find omega-3 and omega-9 fatty acids mostly in the 2, 3, 4, and 7B food groups, and antioxidants in groups 6, 7A, 7B, 8 and 9.

1. **Protein (white is best)**
   - Fish, any
   - Egg whites, Egg Beaters
   - Chicken and turkey, lean
   - Tofu
   - Fat-free cottage cheese
   - Daily omega-3/free range whole egg

2. **Fish**
   - Oily fish, e.g., salmon, sardines, tuna, herring, mackerel, anchovies, cod, trout, bluefish, e.g., halibut, occasional swordfish
   - Canned fish

Fresh fish is better than canned, raw fish is better than cooked, and wild fish are better than farmed.

Fish Contamination

As you may be aware, fish may be contaminated with mercury and other toxic substances. I don't have a clear answer about how to prevent and avoid mercury contamination. I eat fish, but I am careful. I read labels and ask questions. Find out where the fish comes from, and do research to remain informed on the latest findings. For more information, see the sidebar on p. 120.

3. Olive oil and olives

- Extra virgin olive oil – cold pressed is best. The highest quality olive oils have a darker residue or sediment, usually on the bottom of the glass container. No other oil is allowed (except flaxseed oil, or fish oil as a supplement).

4. Nuts and flaxseed oil

- Walnuts are best, though macadamias, pumpkin seeds, almonds, and hazelnuts are acceptable
- NO peanuts, cashews, Brazil nuts, pecans or foods made from them
- Walnut oil is also acceptable on occasion

5. Grains, pulses and beans

- Rice
- Brown rice
- Lentils
- Beans (canned OK)
- Greens/string beans
- Peas and chickpeas only a bit, on occasion
- NO Corn

6. Wine

- Red wine only, 2-4 oz, with dinner only. Red wine is the only wine on this diet, and only at dinner. Start once a week, at home, and then talk to your doctor. No driving, and be aware of side effects. This is strongly discouraged for people with histories of alcohol abuse or intolerance.

7A. Vegetables

- Fresh vegetables (a variety of classifications and colors) are best, ideally eaten raw
- Frozen vegetables are acceptable, as are steamed and cooked vegetables
- Omega-3 green leafy vegetables (see next group) are even better

7B. Omega-3 vegetables

- Spinach
- Arugula
- Lettuces
- Kale
- Collard greens
- Alfalfa sprouts
- Broccoli
- Watercress
- Mustard greens
- Cauliflower
- Bean sprouts

8. Raw fruit

- Eat a variety of fruits, ideally only those in season and already ripened when picked.

9. Herbs

- Fresh: Get them in bags at the market, in pots from a home store, or from your garden.
- Dry: bay leaves, coriander, ground cumin, dill, garlic, oregano, rosemary, tarragon, thyme, etc.

10. Banned foods from the above categories

Eat NO corn, potatoes, flour, fried food or meat. Dairy products are also to be avoided, but a little on rare occasions is acceptable.

For a more detailed description of the Jupiter Institute Omega Diet, turn to page 99 or visit our website (www.jupiterinstitute.com).

WHAT NOT TO EAT: FOUR ENEMIES

Each one of these following five "enemies" would need a whole chapter to be explained. Since weight loss is not the primary purpose of this book, my presentation here is condensed, but we advise you to read and re-read the following sections: these five "bad guys" need to be identified and remembered.

1. **Energy-dense or calorie-dense food**

   This group consists of manufactured "foods" concentrating a large amount of calories in small volume items: candy bars, cakes, shakes, desserts, pizza, fast food, artificial drinks, chocolate, cookies, packed snacks and more. All of these have been created to look appealing and taste delicious. They are unhealthy because they are very high in concentrated calories. They are made by mixing high-calorie ingredients (sugar, fat, butter, syrups, chocolate, peanuts, etc.) to make a small product very dense in calories, and hence very fattening. Picture this: one Snickers' bar has almost 300 calories, nearly one-quarter of your daily caloric intake. Now, think how quickly you can eat one bar. Those calories add up, and the body converts them into fat and stores them in our cells.

   Some natural foods are also calorie-dense, e.g., oils and fatty meats like bacon.

2. **High-caloric meals and snacks**

   Every time we eat a meal with an excessive amount of calories, if the amount of calories ingested is greater than the calories needed for our physical activity, the excess calories are converted into fat. So, the ridiculously huge portions served in restaurants, meals prepared with high-calorie additives such as oil, brown sugar, bacon, lard, molasses and butter, and unnecessary snacking or emotional eating are fat-creating habits. Additionally, it matters not whether the excess calories are in the form of proteins, fats or carbohydrates. Remember the Snickers bar? If we eat it after we have already eaten the amount of daily calories we need, all the calories in that bar will go straight to our fat stores.

Good examples of high-calorie meals are pasta with store-bought tomato sauce and meatballs, which combine excessive amount of processed carbohydrates (the pasta) with lots of fat and oil; or a double cheeseburger, which has heavy concentrations of fats, lard, oils and carbohydrates; or a feast of ribs and chips. Other examples of high calorie meals include large servings of home-made fried chicken; meat and potatoes; corn, mashed potatoes, and meat loaf with gravy; turkey with stuffing, pie, gravy and trimmings; and a breakfast feast of cereal with milk and a bagel with cream cheese, with juice and eggs.

3. **Processed carbohydrates and fat-free foods**
   Processed carbohydrates are carbohydrates altered by manufacturing: "pre-digested," simplified, and made easy to eat. Processing destroys the natural structure of the food and a great deal of its original nutritional value. While processed foods can be easy to digest and absorb, they also contain chemicals and additives that affect human metabolism and cause weight gain. These foods are absorbed fast, and quickly converted into fat. Some examples:

   • From corn: muffins, chips, tortillas, tacos, cereal
   • From potatoes: mashed potatoes, chips, French fries
   • From wheat: bread, crackers, cakes, pasta, cereal
   • From fruits: juices of all kind

Foods that claim to be "fat-free" also mislead us. Generally, these foods are laden with sugars, and have a tendency to make us want more of the product. Unfortunately, fat-free does not mean "Free Ride!"

4. Processed food (a.k.a. factory food)

Most processed foods are made in appealing colors and with enhanced flavors. They combine processed carbohydrates, processed fats, factory-made oils (the worst of the edible oils – also known as trans fats or trans fatty acids), chemicals, colorants and flavor enhancers. They look great and taste better but don't be fooled. They have been ground, cooked, fried and baked, and the food's natural structure has been destroyed in the process. They also have a variety of additives that make you want to eat more. Because the processing has "pre-digested" them, your system digests them so quickly that the blood stream is flooded with large amounts of glucose, causing insulin reaction and weight gain.

These four food groups (1, 2, 3 and 4) are dangerous because they promote weight gain, but they are especially so because they all contain either omega-6 fatty acids, are activators of omega-6s, or are stimulators of harmful eicosanoids. Simply put, they cause inflammation. The more you eat them, the farther they push you into an unhealthy state.

Our Toxic Nutritional Environment

Our prevailing culture encourages us to take in excessive, unnecessary energy in the form of calories from:

- easily available and abundant energy-dense, high-fat and processed foods
- high-calorie meals and huge portions, at home and in restaurants
- smart advertising and misleading marketing
- fancy labels and seductive packaging
- the habit of snacking

These factors, along with our sedentary lifestyles, have produced a toxic environment, a "pro-inflammatory" nutritional condition that promotes disease and illness.

MORE ABOUT PROCESSED CARBOHYDRATES

As I have said, processed carbohydrates (carbs) are appetite-enhancers, tasty to eat and temporarily satisfying, but their effect on blood glucose and insulin causes rebound hunger. Depending on the amount and types of carbohydrates and the kind of processing they have undergone, this rebound hunger may be felt in as little as a half-hour or as much as two hours. But when it hits you will want to eat more.

The larger the amount of carbohydrates and the more processed they are, the higher the blood sugar response and the stronger the rebound hunger. The stronger the hunger, the more control you lose, the more you eat and the more weight you gain. That is why simple carbohydrates are dangerous.

Excess and processed carbs in general are dangerous for other reasons as well. They stimulate the omega-6 path, pushing you into the omega-6/free-radical state, making it difficult to lose weight and, once lost, easy to regain it.

Carbs are also destructive because they trigger an excessive secretion of insulin, which leads to an almost immediate conversion of carbs into fat. Yes, just like that: excess carbohydrates cause excess fat.

These are extremely important concepts for effective weight management, so understand them well. We live in a dangerously high-carbohydrate society, and we are surrounded by unhealthy carbs wherever we go. For these reasons, processed carbohydrates are not permitted during the weight-loss phase where we are focused on eliminating inflammation through food choices. Here are some examples of forbidden carbs:

- From grains and pulses: rice products (rice cakes, rice crackers), bean products (dips, refried beans), green peas, and corn products (chips, soups, corn bread, muffins, anything made with cornstarch or corn meal), wheat and wheat products (flour products, bread, pasta, cakes, muffins, crackers, bagels, and donuts). However, you will be able to enjoy unprocessed rice, lentils and beans in certain specified meals taken during this phase.

- Oatmeal and cereal, including ALL commercial cereals.
- Tubers: potato, mashed potato; mashed yams and sweet potato.
- Any fruit juice or jelly; canned sodas.
- Sweets: candies, dessert, bars, snacks, ice cream, sherbet.
- Diet bars and food sold as "diet" food.
- Alcohol: beer, liquor and any alcoholic beverages except red wine.
- Fast food and "junk-food" frozen dinners; all are loaded with excess carbohydrates.

PROCESSED CARBOHYDRATES ARE AGENTS OF OBESITY, DISEASE AND INFLAMMATION

To sum up, processed carbohydrates are dangerous for three main reasons:

1. They cause rebound hunger, which we've just described, so you wind up eating again in 1-2 hours. Those extra calories push you toward obesity.

2. Excess carbohydrates trigger an insulin reaction that quickly converts a large portion of carbohydrates into fat. This increases weight, increases the fat in the bloodstream (causing hyperlipidemia and atherosclerosis), and is the activity that promotes Type 2 diabetes.

3. Processed carbohydrates stimulate the omega-6/negative-eicosanoid pathway, which promotes inflammation, interferes with weight loss, and may actually cause weight gain.

These are the three main causes of obesity in this country. Think about it: the country's overabundance of carbohydrates is overwhelming. Whether we are at home, work, the mall or the movies, we are always surrounded by carbohydrates. I cannot emphasize enough how critical it is to understand these concepts, especially if you suffer from obesity, diabetes or cardiovascular disease.

RULES

As you prepare your food, follow these rules:

1. **Nothing fried.** Sauté using a Teflon pan, and use a tablespoon of broth to help you sauté. While high-quality oil sprays – which can be found at your local health food store – can be used, they are discouraged. Cooked oils are proven carcinogens. Additionally, they inhibit the body's ability to absorb nutrients.

2. **Never use oil for cooking.** Use Extra Virgin olive oil only for uncooked sauces and dressings.

3. **You must eat essential fats.** There are very important nutrients (a.k.a. essential fatty acids and omega fatty acids) found in some nuts (mainly walnuts), olive oil, flaxseed oil, fish, fish oil, salmon oil and green leafy vegetables. For the best types of fish and vegetables see the lists on pages 113 & 117. A lack of omega fatty acids can cause nutritional deficiencies, illnesses, and bad metabolism; it can also prevent weight loss, cause weight gain, and endanger your health. Fat-free diets and very low-fat diets are strongly discouraged because they are devoid of these important nutrients.

4. **Make your meals tasty.** Avoid boredom. Boredom and monotony jeopardize dieting efforts.

5. **Don't skip meals:** skipping meals is a cause of obesity. It is a myth that avoiding breakfast or lunch helps you lose weight. On the contrary, it makes you gain weight. Overweight people have slower metabolism. Skipping meals slows metabolism even more. Food and exercise are natural metabolism accelerators. Never skip breakfast. Never skip lunch.

6. **Be disciplined:** plan your meals ahead, surround yourself with the food you are allowed to eat, and get into the habit of eating only when suggested without snacking in between meals.

7. **Do not eat "forbidden carbs,"** and remember the four enemies.

8. **Plan your meals.** Don't wait until you are hungry to decide what you are going to eat or your hunger will decide for you.

9. **Remember FaFa (Fa**ctory food is **Fa**ttening food). Learn the difference between factory foods and natural foods.

10. **Protein consumption** is mandatory to prevent "auto-cannibalization," which occurs when the body devours its own muscles. You must eat the indicated amount and even supplement it on exercise days.

11. **Olive oil for breakfast.** Yes. This is very important. It is part of the program. You can improve the flavor with a bit of "I can't believe it's not butter," mustard, fat-free mayonnaise, ketchup, herbs or seasonings. If you are having something savory, add a touch of olive oil for health.

12. **Essential oils** (flaxseed, olive, fish/salmon), either liquid or in the supplement form of gel caps, are not to be missed.

13. **Diet bars** are dangerous to this and every diet. Stay away from them. (Remember: factory food is fattening food).

14. **Sea salt** contains better minerals than regular iodized salt. Use only sea salt, and minimally.

15. **On heavy exercise days** you need more protein. Add either 2 eggs or ½ cup of cottage cheese, or 1 cup of Egg-Beaters or 3 ounces of tuna to your meal, either at dinner or the following breakfast.

16. **You can't substitute for nature.** Fresh vegetables, fruits and herbs provide essential nutrients that pills can't replace. Consume them as instructed.

17. **Vitamins, calcium and other supplements, minerals and non-prescription pills** are not permitted unless approved by the doctor monitoring your diet.

18. **Don't plan your weekend entertainment around food,** unless you know you will be able to stick with the rules!

Feeling unwell? Tired? Achy? Dizzy? Crabby? Cramps? Try 1 cup of bouillon, get some rest, and call your doctor if you still don't feel well.

For medical questions and concerns, call your primary care doctor.

NARROWING YOUR ENVIRONMENT

Imagine yourself at a vegetables-only buffet and then transport yourself to a pasta-and-seafood buffet. Or, think of yourself in a house with only beans, veggies, chicken and fruits, and then in another home full of a large variety of snacks and desserts. The latter of both examples exposes you to a larger amount of more delicious foods. They give you more choices, make your life easier, provide more satisfaction, and make you eat more and gain weight! So, are they really easier and more satisfying?

The more often you are exposed to an environment full of attractive food, the more difficult it will be for you to lose weight and to keep it off. Elaborate brunches or week-long vacation cruises broaden your food environment and are dangerous for anyone on a diet plan.

Limiting the variety and quantity of available foods is crucial in weight loss and maintenance programs.

People in the weight-management phase may be able to control the amount and types of food they consume if the food stimuli to which they are exposed are controlled or limited. We will call this concept "narrowing your food environment." Remember to observe this concept throughout your program.

If you have a weight problem, narrow your food environment. The suggested menus in the next section will help you do this.

WEIGHT-LOSS DIET MENU CHOICES
Breakfast Options (Approx. 220 Cal)

Choose one of the following:

- ½ cup of Egg Beaters (with olive oil spray on Teflon pan when you sauté)
- ½ cup of fresh berries or fruit, mixed with 6-oz. size cup of fat-free plain yogurt (soy yogurt is permitted occasionally) or ½ cup of fat-free cottage cheese
- 1 egg scrambled on Teflon, with olive oil spray, 1 cup of chopped raw vegetables (either sautéed with the egg or separated). Veggies must be crunchy every time you sauté them. Omega-3 and free-range eggs are preferred, and 1 cup of fresh berries or fruits
- ⅔ cup of Egg Beaters sautéed in olive oil spray on Teflon with either 1 cup of chopped vegetables or raw spinach (2 bags of 20-calorie or 1 bag of 40-calorie). Veggies must be crunchy every time you sauté them: 1 cup of fruit is allowed
- Cottage cheese (1 small 4-oz. snack size, or ⅓ cup fat-free or 2%) mixed with 2 tablespoons of fat-free sour cream and 1 cup of chopped vegetables, or ½ cup of fruit

- Cottage cheese (¾ cup fat-free or 2%) with 1 tablespoon of fat-free sour cream, mixed with one cup of chopped vegetables
- Cottage cheese (⅔ cup fat-free or 2%) mixed with 1 cup chopped fruit or berries. Optional: 1 tablespoon of either fat-free sour cream or fat-free plain yogurt
- 1 boiled egg, ½ cup fat-free cottage cheese – omega-3 and free-range eggs are preferred
- 6 egg whites, scrambled with 1 cup of chopped vegetables or 1 bag (40 calories) of spinach, and ½ cup of fruit
- 1 Optifast® shake
- 7 egg whites, or 1 full cup of Egg Beaters, scrambled in olive oil spray on Teflon with 1½ cup of chopped vegetables
- 1 egg or ⅔ cup of Egg Beaters sautéed with 1 can of mushrooms, green beans or asparagus, and ½ cup of fruit
- 2 eggs boiled, with 1 teaspoon of mustard or ketchup and ½ cup of fruit

NOTES:

✦ Add either ½ teaspoon of ground/minced walnut, or 1 teaspoon of olive oil to your breakfast choice, or use one of the sauce choices in Chapter 11.
✦ When you sauté, always use a Teflon pan and olive oil spray only.
✦ For other meal choices: read the substitution list in this chapter.
✦ See the vegetables list on the next page: Only listed vegetables are permitted.
✦ Feel free to use sea salt (unless contraindicated), seasonings and herbs to assure the good taste of your meal. Walnut and olive oil are highly recommended.
✦ Breakfast in the car is forbidden, as is skipping breakfast.
✦ Supplements: 2 gel caps of salmon oil.

BREAKFAST DRINKS

- Decaf coffee with a little fat-free milk, or
- Herbal tea, or
- Instant coffee (made with ½ teaspoon of instant coffee and a little fat-free milk)

Midday Snack (approx. 80 cal)

The timing of this snack depends on your schedule. Midday means mid-morning for some, and mid-afternoon for others. The choices are:

- 1 hard-boiled egg, with sauce from list in Chapter 11.
- ¾ cup of fat-free plain yogurt or sauce (see sauces later in this chapter), fat-free cottage cheese, with stevia (herbal sweetener) and ½ teaspoon of walnut or olive oil.
- 1 cup of fresh fruit and 2 tablespoons of cottage cheese, fat-free or 2%.
- 2 roll-ups. Each roll-up made with 4 leaves of lettuce, 1 slice of chicken or turkey cold-cut.
- 1⅓ cup of chopped vegetables with two tablespoons of fat-free sour cream or yogurt or cottage cheese, and a no-calorie drink.

If you prefer other choices, discuss them with your doctor.

This snack is part of the program. Arrange your schedule so you can take the time to have it. Once you set the time for this snack, stick to it. Always eat at the same time.

Always plan your meals ahead of time and surround yourself with foods you are allowed to eat. Avoid exposure to foods that are not permitted on the plan. Avoid skipping meals: you will be hungry later and may lose control over your plan.

Vegetables And Morning Vegetables

Alfalfa sprouts*

Arugula*

Asparagus

Bean sprouts*

Broccoli*

Cabbage

Cauliflower*

Celery

Chives

Collard greens*

Cucumber

Garlic

Kale*

Lettuce

Mushrooms

Mustard greens*

Onions

Peppers

Romaine lettuce

Scallions

Snow peas

Spinach

Swiss chard*

Tomato

Watercress*

Zucchini

Those marked * provide omega-3s and are the best for you.

Bits of bamboo shoots, and canned mushrooms or asparagus are OK.

As you can see, potatoes, yams and sweet potatoes are forbidden.

Raw carrots, green peas and snap peas are higher in calories, so you may use only a little, as an additive.

Thawed frozen vegetables are allowed only in small amounts to garnish your salad.

Free Use

- Fresh herbs are strongly encouraged: basil, chives, cilantro, dill, garlic, ginger, parsley, rosemary, thyme. Buy them in bags or in pots. Grow them in your garden. Add them to your salad whenever possible.
- Dry herbs and seasonings: anything you like from the supermarket shelf.
- Flavoring: lemon and lime juice, salt, sea salt, vinegar, balsamic vinegar, black pepper, garlic powder.

Dinner (approx. 530 cal)
Choose one protein
**best   *second best*

- *Chicken breast, no skin, no fat, 1½ size of your palm, baked, grilled or roasted. Free-range preferred.
- Chicken, Tyson's tray for example, either 2 breasts or 4 drumsticks, no skin, no juice.
- Shrimp, 14 large or 25 medium size (neither extra-large nor small salad type), grilled or boiled.
- Steak, lean or grilled, 1½ size of your palm.
- *Fish, white meat, 1½ whole-hand size, (cod, grouper, snapper, tilapia, mahi-mahi, catfish, flounder, etc.), baked or grilled.
- Cold cuts, ¾ lb of turkey or chicken, or 9 hand-shaped slices of pastrami, or roast beef, medium-slice cut.

- *Turkey, lean, white meat, 2 palm-size portions.
- *Eggs, 4, scrambled with Olive Oil Spray on Teflon. Free-range/omega preferred.
- *Egg beaters, 2½ cups, with Olive Oil Spray on Teflon.
- **Fresh tuna, salmon or mackerel, 1½ palm-size portion, grilled or poached. On occasion, swordfish (1½ palm size) or halibut (1¾ palm size).
- **Canned tuna or salmon in water, one 6-ounce can and one 3-ounce can.
- *Cottage cheese, fat-free or 2%, 1¾ cups. Add 1-2 tablespoons of sauce to your choice.

Pick one dinner salad
- Tossed salad, 6 cups.
- Arugula and lettuce salad, full medium bowl.
- Any combination of the vegetable list, 6 cups.
- Mixed green vegetables, full small bowl.
- Whole cauliflower or broccoli, raw or steamed.

Dress your salad with a dressing made with 2 teaspoons of oil, or 1 teaspoon of oil and 1 teaspoon of nuts (crushed/sliced/chopped).

Beverage options
Have a no-calorie drink of your choice.

SUBSTITUTIONS

Once or twice a week (but not on exercise days) you may replace one-half of your protein serving by adding one of the following to your salad:

- 2 generous tablespoons of walnuts
- 4 additional teaspoons of oil
- 1 tablespoon of walnuts and 2 teaspoons of oil

You may also replace one-half of your salad with a piece of fruit or 1 cup of chopped fruits, berries or grapes.

Walnuts, fruits and olive oil provide important nutrition, so we encourage these substitutions.

ONCE A WEEK DINNER OPTIONS

- Whole can of beans, 4 cups of chopped vegetables and dressing made with 1 teaspoon of oil.
- ½ of the protein serving, and 1½ cup of rice, white or brown, or lentils, mixed with 2 tablespoons of bouillon and 1 teaspoon of olive oil. (No salad.)
- Lentils, 3 cups, and chopped vegetables, 3 cups, and dressing made with 2 teaspoons of olive oil.

You may replace your salad with two cans of mushrooms, green beans or asparagus – drain & heat with few tablespoons of bouillon and add 1 teaspoon of oil.

A dinner is a dinner. Don't make all the above substitutions, options and choices in the same week. Maintain some variety.

You must consume all dressing, oil and nuts whenever mentioned, as they provide essential fatty nutrients.

ADDITIONAL DINNER CHOICES

- Tofu choice: 1 whole block of tofu, 4 cups of chopped vegetables, and dressing made with 2 teaspoons of olive oil. Or ½ block of tofu, 8 cups of chopped vegetables, and dressing made with 3 teaspoons of oil.
- Sushi choice: Either 10 pieces of maki sushi (rolls – note: not hand rolls) or 8 pieces of sashimi (just the fish without the sushi rice). (No other food with this dinner.)

DINING OUT

Dining out is discouraged and unsafe on this diet! If you must eat out, do so no more than once a week. Fast food places, buffets, take-outs and "all-you-can-eat" restaurants are forbidden. Meals should be mainly vegetarian. Remember, no restaurant is reliable. Choices:

- 1 baked potato, chef or Caesar salad with no croutons, cheese or dressing
- Thai vegetarian dishes without oil and not fried; 1 cup of rice
- Small steak, plain, no sauce; 2 side salads with salt and lemon
- Chinese Buddha's delight without oil or steamed vegetables; 1 small box of rice
- Japanese sushi, sashimi
- Grilled chicken or fish over salad, with only 2 teaspoons of vinaigrette

WINE OPTION

Red wine only. No other alcohol is allowed. Three times a week you can either:

- substitute 4 ounces of red wine for ½ of the salad, or
- substitute 4 ounces of red wine for ½ of the protein, and add 2 more teaspoons of olive oil to your salad (or 2 generous tablespoons of ground walnuts).

We encourage drinking red wine at least once a week, and only during the meal.

Regardless of any substitution, you must take the prescribed supplements.

On heavy exercise days, you need more protein. Do not substitute for your dinner protein, and you need to add to your dinner 2 eggs (any style), or ½ cup cottage cheese, or a 3-ounce can of tuna or 1 cup of Egg Beaters.

Night Snack (approx. 45 cal)

- Cottage cheese, fat-free, ¼ cup; or ricotta, fat-free, ¼ cup; or fat-free plain yogurt, ½ cup, mixed with sugar substitute and flavoring extract.
- Or a choice of fruit:
  1 cup of cantaloupe, grapes, strawberries or papaya
  1 orange
  ½ mango
  ½ cup of banana or blueberries

Sauces

For your breakfast, lunch and dinner, mix any of the following with one tablespoon of olive oil:

- Fat-free barbecue sauce
- Ketchup
- Dijon mustard
- Fat-free mayonnaise
- Fat-free tartar sauce
- Horseradish sauce
- Hot sauce (Habanero, Tabasco, Crystal, etc.)
- Mustard
- Soy sauce
- Taco sauce
- Worcestershire sauce (Lea & Perrins)

Or try the following combinations with one tablespoon of olive oil.

- Parisienne sauce: ¼ teaspoon of Dijon mustard, 1 teaspoon of fat-free mayonnaise.
- European sauce: ¼ teaspoon of mustard; fat-free mayonnaise and horseradish.
- Golf Sauce: 1 teaspoon ketchup, 1 teaspoon fat-free mayonnaise and ¼ teaspoon of Dijon mustard.
- Hot sauce: 1½ teaspoon ketchup, few drops hot sauce, ½ teaspoon horseradish sauce.

Breakfast sauce – place one teaspoon of olive oil in a cup and mix with any one of the above.

Master the art of using sauces, fresh herbs, dressings and seasonings to add culinary excitement to your eating. Try mixing your olive oil with fat-free plain yogurt, fat-free sour cream, and then adding it to any of the above.

Dressings And Salad Dressings

Our basic salad dressing calls for 4 parts oil, 1 part lemon/lime juice or vinegar, and salt and pepper to taste. This basic dressing is then combined with different herbs and spices to become a delicious sauce or dressing.

Step 1. Basic salad dressing
Pour into a cup or glass:
¼ teaspoon of salt
¼ teaspoon of sugar (or pinch of sugar substitute: better yet use Stevia, an herbal sweetener available at health-food stores)
½-1 teaspoon of either vinegar or lemon or lime juice (optional)
Dash of freshly ground black pepper

Mix well.

NOTE: If using soy sauce, prepare the basic salad dressing without salt.

If you are preparing oriental dressings (Thai, Chinese, Japanese, etc) use rice vinegar. Use lime juice for Mexican, and lemon juice for Italian. For Greek and Mediterranean dressings use balsamic vinegar. Some of the sauces will do better without any lemon/lime or vinegar and you might need to try two or three times before you make it right for you.

Some may prefer it with 1½ teaspoons of lemon juice and Tabasco, while others would rather not to use them. In some you may need more salt. Nevertheless, you must not change or skip the olive oil.

I took these recipes from international cookbooks; some you will like, some you may not.

As you prepare, remember 1 teaspoon = 5 cc = 5 ml; 1 tablespoon = 3 teaspoons = 15 cc.

While you don't need to use exact measurements, measuring spoons give the best results. If using spoons from your flatware collection, use the same style of tablespoons and teaspoons on a daily basis.

Now, add four parts of olive oil (1, 2 or 3 teaspoons). You may substitute for each teaspoon 6 olives (green, black, plain or chopped). On occasion, you may replace 1 teaspoon of the olive oil with ½ tablespoon of ground/minced walnuts (unsalted).

Step 2. Add to the basic salad dressing

Add the following combinations to prepare your dressing of choice, mix it well and let it stand. (The quantity of seasonings in each combination may vary according to taste.)

TO MAKE	ADD
Soy sauce dressing	1 tablespoon soy sauce and 1 teaspoon minced green onion
Mustard dressing	½-1 teaspoon Dijon mustard and 2 teaspoons soy sauce
Curry sauce	¼-½ teaspoon fat-free mayonnaise or plain yogurt and curry powder to taste
Curry-Thai dressing	curry powder, chili powder, hot sauce to taste. (It's OK to add toasted coconut, chopped peanuts, or a bit of chopped cilantro)

In curry, Thai and Panang dressings, you can substitute ground/minced carrot for the sugar or sugar substitute in the Basic Salad Dressing.

TO MAKE	ADD
Ketchup sauce	1 tablespoon ketchup
Chinese dressing	½ tablespoon soy sauce and ½ tablespoon of sake or Mirin cooking wine
Taiwan ginger sauce	½-¾ teaspoon soy sauce and minced ginger to taste
Arabic dressing	1 tablespoon hummus ½ teaspoon tahini ½-1 teaspoon chopped olives pinch of paprika
Mexican dressing	1-2 tablespoons chopped tomatoes, with a bit of chopped garlic, chopped cilantro, chili powder or chopped chilies, ground cumin and onion powder
Jalisco dressing	2 tablespoons chopped green peppers, 1-2 tablespoons chopped tomatoes, 1-2 teaspoons chopped red peppers, 1-3 teaspoons chopped onions chopped fresh cilantro, cumin powder and chili powder or a bit of chopped chilies
Busy-Maria dressing	chili powder with onion powder and cumin powder to taste
Mediterranean dressing	1 tablespoon chopped parsley, with 1 teaspoon of chopped onions, coarsely chopped rosemary and tarragon

TO MAKE	ADD
Mediterranean dressing (2)	chopped parsley, with 1-4 teaspoons chopped green and black olives, ¼-½ teaspoons chopped tomatoes, minced or finely chopped onions, and a pinch each of oregano, thyme and rosemary
Nadine's dressing	extra tablespoon of olive oil pinch of oregano 1½ tablespoon crumbled feta cheese ½ teaspoon lemon juice
Pesto dressing	1-2 tablespoons chopped basil, with ½ teaspoon chopped walnuts and a bit of Parmesan cheese
Teriyaki dressing	½-¾ tablespoon sake ½ tablespoon of Mirin cooking wine 1 teaspoon soy sauce
Popo's dressing	1½ tablespoon of any sauce in a Chinese or Japanese market
Sotogary dressing	2 teaspoon soy sauce ½ teaspoon French mustard ¼ teaspoon minced garlic ¼-¾ teaspoon minced ginger a little minced onion and tamari sauce
Yaya's dressing	1 tablespoon balsamic vinegar with extra olive oil and extra salt; always mix the ingredients well and let the dressing stand for 10 minutes before you try it

TO MAKE	ADD
Kyoto sauce	1-2 teaspoon of soy sauce ½-1 tablespoon Mirin cooking wine ½-1 tablespoon clear broth ¼ teaspoon mustard
Anchovy sauce	1 tablespoon thin chopped anchovies 1-2 teaspoon white wine
Argentinean sauce	½-1 tablespoon dry thyme and oregano pinch of bay leaves powder ½ tablespoon of chopped parsley 1 teaspoon minced garlic
Green sauce	1 tablespoon of thinly chopped green peppers ½ tablespoon thinly chopped anchovies 1 teaspoon chopped parsley 1 teaspoon white wine a drop of water 1-3 teaspoons chopped basil (Some prefer more parsley than basil, some like it the other way around. Be careful; parsley kills the taste of basil. Some like to exchange cilantro for basil. You may try the recipe omitting parsley; mixing basil and cilantro instead.)
Red sauce	1-3 tablespoons chopped tomatoes 1 tablespoon chopped red pepper 1-2 tablespoons red wine pinch of chili powder, pinch of paprika, pinch of cumin powder, pinch of onion powder

TO MAKE	ADD
Northern Greek sauce	1-3 tablespoons of chopped red pepper, with pinch of dry oregano, pinch of coarsely chopped rosemary, 1-3 teaspoon chopped green peppers, 1-4 teaspoons finely chopped anchovies, 1-4 chopped black olives and chopped parsley; you may also add a bit of minced onions or garlic.
Southern Greek sauce	Coarsely chopped rosemary with dry oregano chopped green and black olives tiny chunks of feta cheese tarragon and a bit of thyme
New Orleans sauce	1-2 tablespoons Louisiana Hot Sauce freshly ground hot pepper 1 teaspoon brown sugar 1-2 teaspoons rum, and 1 teaspoon of that seasoning you got as a souvenir
Dry herbal sauce	a pinch of any three of the following: oregano, thyme, tarragon, dill, rosemary, white pepper, freshly ground black pepper, ground bay leaves, marjoram

TO MAKE	ADD
Napoli sauce	1 tablespoon of chopped fresh basil pinch of dry oregano 1 tablespoon finely chopped tomato 3 chopped green olives 1-2 tablespoons finely chopped green pepper bit of minced or finely chopped onion and fresh garlic 1 teaspoon chopped parsley
Thai sauce	1 tablespoon chopped mint leaves 1 tablespoon finely chopped cilantro leaves ½-1 teaspoon minced fresh ginger 1 tablespoon broth
Thai Ginger sauce	½-1 teaspoon of finely chopped or minced fresh ginger 1-2 teaspoons soy sauce 1-2 teaspoons broth 1-3 teaspoons chopped mint leaves Pinch of chili powder (or ½-1 teaspoon of finely chopped chili), hot sauce, and ½ teaspoon curry powder are optional.
Panang sauce	¼ teaspoon of cumin powder ¼-½ teaspoon curry powder pinch of chili powder (or finely chopped ¼-½ tsp of chili) ½ tablespoon chopped cilantro leaves 1-3 teaspoons chopped peanuts, (or 1-2 teaspoons peanut butter) a tiny bit of garlic or onion powder; hot sauce is optional

TO MAKE	ADD
Swiss sauce	1 teaspoon ketchup 1 teaspoon fat-free mayonnaise ½ teaspoon mustard
Dry Sicily sauce	2 teaspoons of white wine a pinch of each: oregano, rosemary and thyme (you may add or exchange for tarragon). On any occasion, you may substitute chopped chives for the onion.
Roma sauce	capers, chopped onions, green peppers, red peppers, basil, parsley and tomato bit of parmesan cheese, drop of white wine
Lorenzo sauce	chili powder and hot sauce
Parisienne sauce	1-3 teaspoons wine of choice
Russian sauce	1 teaspoon horseradish 2 teaspoons ketchup
Krafty sauce	Add 2-3 teaspoons of your choice of fat-free salad dressing
"Easy-ones" sauce	add ½ teaspoon of your choice of: Worcestershire sauce fat-free mayonnaise ketchup taco sauce salsa hot sauce

Variations: Different cooks of different nationalities prepare the same dressings in different ways. Some add more seasonings and herbs, and others may not use the same amount of ingredients that we present on this list. In addition, your own palate and preferences may dictate certain variations to satisfy your own personal taste. Feel free to make changes when preparing these dressings and sauces. **But never skip the olive oil!** And you can always add ¼-½ teaspoon more olive oil if the dressing or sauce turns out too thick. On occasion, however, you may – if you dare – substitute salmon or fish oil for the olive oil. I have done so a few times, adding it to salmon or salads, and I liked the result. My wife Ana, however, refuses to go near it.

You can use the olive oil as a sauce with your protein. In this case don't use the olive oil for your salad (just have your salad with lemon juice, salt, herbs or with a bit of fat-free mayonnaise). Then prepare the sauce (for your protein) mixing the ingredients from the above pages, and the olive oil, and adding vinegar or lemon juice as you please.

If there is another sauce or dressing you want to suggest, fax, mail or e-mail it to me. I may post it on my website and share it with my patients.

APPENDICES:
RESOURCES FOR YOUR HEALTH

The following is a list of organizations and sources of information that readers may contact.

PAIN

American Academy of Pain Management
Sonora, California
Tel.: (209) 533-9744 – Fax: (209) 533-9750
www.aapainmanage.org

American Academy of Pain Medicine
Glenview, IL
www.painmed.org

The American Chronic Pain Association
Rocklin, California
Tel.: (916) 632-0922 – Fax: (916) 632-3208
www.theacpa.org

The American Pain Society
Glenview, Illinois
Tel.: (847) 375-4715 – Fax: (847) 375-6315
www.ampainsoc.org

International Association for the Study of Pain
Seattle, Washington
Tel.: (206) 547-6409 – Fax: (206) 547-1703
www.halcyon.com
www.iasp-pain.org

The American Pain Foundation
Baltimore, Maryland
www.painfoundation.org

The National Foundation for the Treatment of Pain
Monterey, California
Tel.: (831) 655-8812 – Fax: (831) 655-2823
www.paincare.org

National Pain Foundation
Denver, Colorado
www.painconnection.org

The Arthritis Foundation
Atlanta, Georgia
Tel.: 1-800-283-7800
www.arthritis.org

Fibromyalgia Network
Tucson, Arizona
Tel.: (520) 290-5508
www.fmnetnews.com

Neuropathy Association
New York, NY
www.neuropathy.org

MEDICAL

American Academy of Craniofacial Pain
www.aacfp.org

American College of Rheumatology
Atlanta, Georgia
Tel.: (404) 633-3777 – Fax: (404) 633-1870
www.rheumatology.org

American Fibromyalgia Syndrome Association
Tucson, AZ
www.afsafund.org

American Headache Society
Mount Royal, NJ
www.ahsnet.org

American Physical Therapy Association
Alexandria, VA
www.apta.org

American Society of Clinical Nutrition
Bethesda, MD
www.faseb.org

The Arthritis Society Toronto, Ontario, Canada
www.arthritis.ca

Food and Drug Administration
Rockville, MD
Tel.: 1-800-532-4440
www.fda.gov

FDA Center for Food Safety and Applied Nutrition
www.cfsan.fda.gov

Mayo Clinic Health Information
www.mayoclinic.com

National Center for Complementary and Alternative Medicine
Tel.: 1-888-644-6226
www.nccam.nih.gov

The National Institutes of Health
Bethesda, MD
www.nih.gov

National Library of Medicine
www.nlm.nih.gov

National Headache Foundation
Chicago, IL
www.headaches.org

World Health Organization
www.who.org

ALTERNATIVE MEDICINE

American Academy of Medical Acupuncture
Los Angeles, California
Tel.: (213) 937-5514 Tel.: (323) 937-5514
Tel.: 1-800-521-AAMA
www.medicalacupuncture.org

American Chiropractic Association
Arlington, VA
Tel.: (703) 276-8800
www.americhiro.org

American Association of Alternative medicine
www.aaom.org

American Massage Therapy Association
Evanston, IL
www.amtamassage.org

American Osteopathic Association
Chicago, IL
www.am-osteo-assn.org

Insight Meditation Society Barre, MA
www.dharma.org

International Chiropractors Association
Arlington, VA
Tel.: 1-800-423-4690
www.chiropractic.org

Mind-Body Medical Institute
Boston, MA
Tel.: (617) 632-9530
www.mindbody.harvard.edu

National Acupuncture and Oriental Medicine Alliance
Olalla, WA
Tel.: (253)851-6896
www.acuall.org

The National Center of Homeopathy
www.homeopathic.org

National Certification Commission for Acupuncture and Oriental
Medicine Alexandria, VA
www.nccoam.org

The Qigong Institute
www.healthy.net

Transcendental Meditation
www.tm.org

More information about acupuncture:
www.acupuncture.com
www.acsh.org
www.healthy.net

HERBAL MEDICINE

American Botanical Council Austin, Texas
www.herbalgram.org
www.herbs.org
www.ahpa.org
www.ars-grin.gov/duke
www.amfoundation.org
www.nutraceuticalinstitute.com
www.medherb.com

NATUROPATHY

American Association of Naturopathic Physicians
Seattle, WA
Tel.: (206) 298-0126
www.naturopathic.org

American Association of Oriental Medicine
Catasaugua, PA
Tel.: 1-888-500-7999 Tel.: (610) 266-1433
www.aaom.org

American Chiropractic Association
Arlington, VA
Tel.: (703) 276-8800 Tel.:1-800-986-4636
www.americhiro.org

SCHOOLS OF NATUROPATHY

Bastyr University
Kenmore, WA
Tel.: (425) 823-1300
www.bastyr.edu

National College of Naturopathic Medicine
Portland, Oregon Tel.: (503) 499-4343
www.ncnm.edu

Southwest College of Naturopathic Medicine
Tempe, Arizona
Tel.: (602) 858-9100
www.scnm.edu

REFERENCES

Adebowale, A.O., and Cox, D.S. "Analysis of glucosamine and chondroitin Sulfate content in marketed products." *Journal of the American Nutraceuticals Association*, 3(1),2000, p37-44.

Aker, P.D., and McDermaid, C. "Searching chiropractic literature: a comparison of three computerized databases" *Journal of Manipulative and Physiological Therapeutics*, Oct. 1996; 19(8):518-24.

Albert, C.M. "Fish consumption and risk of sudden cardiac death." *Journal of the American Medical Association*, 1998, 279:23-28.

Arnold, W., and Berman, B. *Arthritis Foundation Guide to Alternative Therapies*. Arthritis Foundation Publications, 2001.

Assendelft, W.J. "The efficacy of chiropractic manipulation for back pain." *Journal of Manipulative and Physiological Therapeutics*, 1992, October, 15(8):487-494.

Audette, J.F., and Ryan, A.H. "The role of acupuncture in pain management." *Physical Medicine and Rehabilitation Clinics of North America*, 2004, 15(4):749-72.

Backonja, M.M. "Neuropathic Pain Syndromes." *Neurologic Clinics*, 1998, 16(4):775-988.

Balch, J.F., and Balch, A.B. *Prescription for Nutritional Healing*. Avery Publishing Group, 1996.

Balch, J.F., and Stengler, M. *Prescription for Natural Cures*. John Wiley and Sons, 1999.

Barnard, Neal D. *Foods That Fight Pain*. Three Rivers Press. 1999. Barney, P. *Doctor's Guide to Natural Medicine*. Woodland Publishing. 1998.

Berman, B.M., and Lao, L. "Effectiveness of acupuncture as adjunctive therapy in osteoarthritis of the knee." *Annals of Internal Medicine*, 2004, Dec, 141(12):901-10.

Bove, G., and Nilsson, N. "Spinal manipulation in the treatment of episodic tension-type headache." *Journal of the American Medical Association*, 1998, Nov, 280(18):1576-79.

Brandt, K.D., and Doherty, M. *Osteoarthritis*. Oxford University Press, 1998.

Bresler, David E. *Free Yourself From Pain*. Awareness Press. 1979. Carey, T.S., and Evans, A.T. "Acute severe low back pain." *Spine*, 1996, Feb. 1;21(3):339-44.

Cassidy, C. "Chinese Medicine users in the United States." *Journal of Alternative and Complementary Medicine,* 4(1):17-27, 1998.

Caudill, M.A. *Managing Pain Before It Manages You*. The Guilford Press, 2001.

Challem, Jack. *The Inflammation Syndrome*, Wiley Publishers. 2003.

Cloutier, M. and Adamson, E. *The Mediterranean Diet*. Avon Books, 2003.

Cochran, Robert T. *Understanding Chronic Pain*. Hillsboro Press. 2007.

Coggon, D., and Reading, I. "Knee Osteoarthritis and Obesity." *International Journal of Obesity and Related Metabolic Disorders*, 2001, 25(5): 622-629.

Credit, L.P., and Hartunian, S.G. *Relieving Sciatica*. Avery Publishing Group, 1999.

Cummings, A. "Glucosamine in Osteoarthritis." *Lancet,* 354 (1999): 1640-1641.

Curtis, B., and O'Keeffe, J. "Understanding the Mediterranean Diet." *Postgraduate Medicine Online*, Vol. 112, August 2002.

Dabbs, V., and Lauretti, W.J. "A risk assessment of cervical manipulation vs. NSAIDs for the treatment of neck pain." *Journal of Manipulative and Physiological Therapeutics*, 1995, 18(8):530-536.

Dalen, J.E. "Conventional and unconventional medicine." *Archives of Internal Medicine*, 1998, 158:2179-81.

Darlington, L.G. "Dietary therapy for arthritis." *Rheumatic Disease Clinics of North America*, 1991, 17:273- 97.

Diehl, D.L., and Kaplan, G. "Use of Acupuncture by American Physicians." *Journal of Alternative and Complementary Medicine*, 3(2):119-126, 1997.

Dillard, J. *The Chronic Pain Solution*. Bantam Books, 2001.

Donati, Stella. *The Great Book of Mediterranean Cuisine*. Chartwell Books, Inc. 2001.

Drum, David. *The Chronic Pain Management Source Book*. Publishing Group, Inc. 1999.

Eaton, S.B., and Konner, M., "Paleolithic nutrition: A consideration of its nature and current implications." *New England Journal of Medicine*, 312:283-89, Jan. 31,1983.

Eisenberg, D. "Integrating Complementary Therapies into Clinical Practice." Harvard Medical School Department of Continuing Education, March 2003.

Felson, D.T., and Anderson, J.J. "Obesity and Knee Osteoarthritis: The Framingham Study." *Annals of Internal Medicine, 1988*, 109(1): 18-24.

Ferro-Luzzi, A., and Branca, F., "Mediterranean Diet, Italian Style." *The American Journal of Clinical Nutrition*, 61:1338S-1345S, 1995.

Fisher, Helen, and Thompson, Cynthia. *The Mediterranean Diet*. Perseus Publishing. 2001.

Fleming, R.M. *Stop Inflammation Now*. Avery-Penguin Group, 2004.

Fontanarosa, P.B., and Lundberg, G.D. "Alternative medicine meets science." *Journal of the American Medical Association*, 1998, 280: 1618-19.

Ford, Norman D. *Painstoppers: The Magic of All Natural Pain Relief*, Parker Publishing. 1994.

Fugh-Berman, A. *Alternative Medicine: What Works*. William & Wilkins, 1997.

Fuhrman, B., and Lavy, A. "Consumption of red wine with meals reduces the susceptibility of human plasma and LDL to lipid oxidation." *The American Journal of Clinical Nutrition*, 1995, 61:549-554.

Garcia-Closas, R., and Serra-Majem, L. "Fish Consumption, Omega-3 Fatty Acids and the Mediterranean Diet." *European Journal of Clinical Nutrition*, 1993, 47:S85-S90.

Germain, B.F. *Osteoarthritis and Musculoskeletal Pain Syndromes*. Appleton & Lange, 1983.

Gordon, G. *The Omega-3 Miracle*. Freedom Press, 2000.

Gordon, Neil F. *Arthritis: Your Complete Exercise Guide*. Human Kinetics. 1993.

Gore, M. *The Arthritis Book*. Allan and Unwin, 1997.

Green S, Buchbinder R, "Acupuncture for Shoulder Pain", *Cochrane Database of Systematic Reviews,* 2005. April; (2): CD005319.

Greenberg, D. *Clinical Neurology*. Appleton and Lange, 1993.

Griffin, M. "Practical Management of Osteoarthritis." *Archives of Family Medicine*, 1995, Dec, 4:1049-1055.

Heine, H. "Structure of Acupuncture Points." *Journal of Traditional Chinese Medicine*, 1988, 8(3): 207-212.

Hiesiger, Emile. *Your Pain is Real*. Regan Books. 2001.

Hochschuler, S., and Reznik, B. *Treat Your Back Without Surgery*. Hunter House Publishers, 1998.

Hollon, M.F. "Direct-to-consumer marketing of prescriptions drugs." *Journal of the American Medical Association*, 281 (1999): 382-384.

Holman, R.T. "Significance of Essential Fatty Acids in Human Nutrition." *Lipids* 1:215, 1976.

Holt, Stephen. *Combat Syndrome X, Y and Z*. Wellness Publishing. 2002.

Hooper, L., and Ness, A.R. "Antioxidant strategy." *Lancet*, 2001, 357: 1705.

Hunder, Gene G. *Mayo Clinic on Arthritis*. Mason Crest Publishers. 2002.

Ianucci, L., and Horowitz, M. *The Unofficial Guide to Overcoming Arthritis*. Macmillan, 1999.

Iso, H. "Intake of fish and omega-3 fatty acids and risk of stroke in women." *Journal of the American Medical Association*, 2001, 285: 304-312.

Jarvis K.B., Phillips, R.B., et al. "Cost per case comparison of back injury claims of chiropractic versus medical management for conditions with identical diagnosis codes." *Journal of Occupational Health,* 33(8);347-852, 1991.

Jenkins, Nancy H. *The Mediterranean Diet Cookbook*. Bantam, 1994.

Jenkins, Nancy H. *The Essential Mediterranean*. Harper & Collins, 2003.

Jonas, W.B., and Levin, J.S. *Essentials of Complementary and Alternative Medicine.* Lippincott William & Wilkins, 1999.

Kahn, H.S. "Wine and mortality." *Annals of Internal Medicine,* Jul 3, 2001; 135(1):66.

Kalauokalani. D., and Cherkin, D.C. "A Comparison of Physician and Nonphysician Acupuncture Treatment for Chronic Low Back Pain." *The Clinical Journal of Pain,* Sep 2005; 21(5):406-11.

Kaptchuk, T. "Acupuncture: Theory, Efficacy and Practice." *Annals of Internal Medicine.* 2002:136:374-383.

Katzenstein, Larry. *Taking Charge of Arthritis.* Reader's Digest Association, 1998.

Kessler, R.C., and Davis, R.B. "Long-term trends in the use of complementary and alternative medical therapies in the United States." *Annals of Internal Medicine,* 2001, 135:262-68.

Keys, A. "Mediterranean Diet and public health." *The American Journal of Clinical Nutrition,* 1995, 61: 1321S-1323S.

Keys, A.B. *How to Eat Well and Stay Well the Mediterranean Way.* Doubleday, 1975.

Killion, K.H., and Kastrup, E.K., editors. *Drugs Facts and Comparisons, 2003.* Wolters Kluwer, 2003.

Klatsky, A.L., and Friedman, G.D. "Wine, liquor, beer and mortality." *American Journal of Epidemiology,* Sep 2003, 58(6): 585-595.

Koes, B.W. "Spinal manipulation for low back pain." *Spine,* 1996, 21(24):2860-2871.

Koopman, William J. "Arthritis and Allied Conditions" in *Textbook of Rheumatology,* William & Wilkins. 1997.

Kriegler, J.S., and Ashenberg, Z.S. "Management of chronic low back pain: a comprehensive approach." *Seminars in Neurology,* 1987, Dec, 7(4): 303-312.

Kris-Etherton, P.M., and Harris, W.S. "Fish Consumption, Fish Oil, omega-3 Fatty Acids, and Cardiovascular Disease." *Circulation*, 2002; 106:2747.

Lane, N.E., and Wallace, D.J. *All About Osteoarthritis*. Oxford University Press, 2002.

Lautenschlager, J. "Acupuncture in treatment of inflammatory rheumatic Disease" *Rheumatology*, 1997; 56: 8-20.

Leskowitz, E. *Complementary and Alternative Medicine in Rehabilitation*. Churchill Livingstone. 2003.

Lesser, M. *Nutrition and Vitamin Therapy*. Grove Press, Inc., 1980.

Levy, A.M., and Fuerst, M.L. *Sports Injury Handbook*. John Wiley and Sons, Inc. 1993.

Liu, Simin. "Mediterranean Diets." *American Journal of Clinical Nutrition*. Vol. 73, No. 4, 847, April 2001.

Lorgeril, M.D., and Salem, P. "Mediterranean Diet, traditional risks factors and the rate of cardiovascular complications." *Circulation*, 1999, 779-85.

Mallon, W. *Orthopaedics for the House Officer*. Williams & Wilkins Company, 1990.

McAlindon, T.E., and LaValley, M.P. "Glucosamine and chondroitin for the treatment of osteoarthritis." *Journal of the American Medical Association*, 2000, 283: 1469-75.

McAlindon, T.E., and Biggee, B.A. "Nutritional Factors and Osteoarthritis." *Current Opinion in Rheumatology*, 2005, Sept.: 17(5):647-52.

Meeker, W.C., and Haldeman, S. "Chiropractic: A Profession at the Crossroads of Mainstream and Alternative Medicine." *Annals of Internal Medicine*, 2002, 136:216-227.

Mercier, L. *Practical Orthopedics*. Mosby, 1991.

Meydani, M., and Natiello, F. "Effect of long-term fish oil supplementation on vitamin E status and lipid peroxidation in women." *The American Journal of Clinical Nutrition*, 1991, 121: 484-491.

Moller, I. "Efficacy of Glucosamine Sulfate in Knee Osteoarthritis." *Arthritis and Rheumatism*, 2005, August 15: 3(4):628-29.

Murray, M., and Pizzorno, J. *Encyclopedia of Natural Medicine.* Prima Publishing, 1998.

Namey, T.C. "Exercise and Arthritis." *Rheumatic Disease Clinics of North America*, 1990, 16(4):791-1023.

Napier, K. *Power Nutrition for Your Chronic Illness.* Macmillan, 2001.

Ness, A.R. "Is olive oil a key ingredient in the Mediterranean Diet?" *International Journal of Epidemiology*, 2002, 31:481-482.

Nestle M., "Mediterranean Diets: Historical and Research Overview." *The American Journal of Clinical Nutrition*, Vol 61, 1313S-1320S, 1995.

Novey, D.W. *Clinician's Complete Reference to Complementary/ Alternative Medicine.* Mosby, 2001.

Osborne, Christine. *Middle Eastern Cooking*, Prion Books, Ltd. 1997.

Panush, R.S. "Nutrition and Rheumatic Disease." *Rheumatic Disease Clinics of North America*, 1991, 17(2): 197-456.

Peirce, A. *A Practical Guide to Natural Medicine.* Stonesong Press. 1999.

Pittler, E.E. "Expert opinions on complementary and alternative therapies for low back pain." *Journal of Manipulative and Physiological Therapeutics*, 1999, 22(2): 87-90.

Pizzorno, J., and Murray, M. *Textbook of Natural Medicine.* Churchill Livingstone, 1999.

Pommeranz, B. "Scientific Research into Acupuncture for the Relief of Pain." *Journal of Alternative and Complementary Medicine,* 2(1):53-60, 1996.

Powles, J. "Commentary: Mediterranean Paradoxes." *International Journal of Epidemiology,* 2001:30:1076-1077, 2001.

Pressman, Alan H., and Shelley, Donna. *Integrative Medicine.* St. Martin Press. 2000.

Raj, Prithvi P. *Pain Medicine: A Comprehensive Review.* Mosby. 1995.

Rakel, R.E., and Bope, E.T. *Conn's Current Therapy.* Saunders, 2003.

Rakel, D. *Integrative Medicine.* Saunders. 2007.

Rao, J.K., and Mihaliak, K. "Use of complementary therapies for arthritis among patients of rheumatologists." *Annals of Internal Medicine,* 1999, 131: 409-16.

Reginster, J.Y., and Deroisy, R. "Long term effects of glucosamine sulphate on osteoarthritis progression." *Lancet,* 357, 2001, 247-48.

Rosenfeld, Arthur. *The Truth About Chronic Pain.* Perseus Books. 2003.

Rudin, D., and Felix, C. *Omega-3 Oils.* Avery Publishing Group, 2000.

Russell, A.S., and Aghazadeh, A.H. "Active ingredient consistency of commercially available glucosamine sulfate." *Journal of Rheumatology,* 29, 2002, 2407-09.

Sandmark, H., and Hogstedt, C. "Osteoarthrosis of the knee in men and women in association with overweight." *Annals of the Rheumatic Diseases,* 1999, 58(3):151-155.

Sarzi-Puttini, P., and Cimmino, M.A. "Osteoarthritis: an Overview of the Disease and its Treatment Strategies." *Seminars in Arthritis and Rheumatism,* 2005 Aug: 35(1):1-10.

Sears, Barry. *The Zone*. Regan Books, 1995.

Shekelle, P.G. "Spinal manipulation for low back pain." Annals of Internal Medicine, 117 (1992): 590-598.

Shils, M. *Modern Nutrition in Health and Disease*. Lea & Febiger, 1994.

Simopolous, A. *The Omega Plan*. Harper Collins, 1998.

Simopoulos, A.P., and Robinson, J. *The Omega Diet*. Harper Perennial. 1999.

Simopoulos, A.P. "Omega-3 fatty acids in health and disease and in growth and development." *The American Journal of Clinical Nutrition,* 54:438-463, 1991.

Simopoulos, A.P., and Herbert, V. *The Eat Well, Be Well Cookbook*. Simon and Schuster, 1986.

Stamatos, John M. *Painbuster*. Henry Holt and Company. 2001. Stenson, W.F. "Dietary supplementation with fish oil in ulcerative colitis." *Annals of Internal Medicine*, 116:609-614, 1992.

Stoddard, D. *Pain Free for Life*. TorchLight Publishing, 1998.

Stoll, Andrew L. *The Omega-3 Connection*. Simon & Schuster. 2001.

The Medical Letter. *The Medical Letter on Drugs and Therapeutics*. The Medical Letter, Inc.

Theodosakis, J. *The Arthritis Cure*. St. Martin Griffin, 2002.

Trichopoulou, A., and Costacou, T. "Adherence to a Mediterranean Diet." *The New England Journal of Medicine*, 348:2599-2608, June 26, 2003.

Vernon, L.F. "Spinal Manipulation as a Valid Treatment for Low Back Pain" *Delaware Medical Journal*, March 1996, 68(3):175-78.

Wall P.D., and Melzack, R. *Textbook of Pain*. Churchill Livingstone, 1999.

Weiger, W. and Smith, M. "Advising patients who seek Complementary and Alternative Medical Therapies." *Annals of Internal Medicine*, 2002:137:889-903.

Weil, A. "Integrated medicine." *British Medical Journal*, 2001, 322: 119-120.

Weil, Andrew. *Eating Well for Optimum Health*. Alfred Knopf Publishers, 2000.

Weil, Andrew. *Health and Healing: Understanding Conventional and Alternative Medicine*. Houghton Mifflin, 1998.

Weinbrenner, T., and Fito, M. "Olive Oils High Phenolic Compounds Modulate Oxidative/ Antioxidative Status in Men." *The American Journal of Clinical Nutrition*, 134-2314-2321, September 2004.

Weiner, R.S. *Pain Management: a Practical Guide for Clinicians*. St. Lucie Press. 1998.

Wiancek, D.A. *The Natural Healing Companion*. Rodale Publishers, 1999.

Willett, W.C., and Sacks, F. "Mediterranean Diet Pyramid: a Cultural Model for Healthy Eating." *The American Journal of Clinical Nutrition*, 61:1402S-1406S, 1995.

Willett, E. *Arthritis*. Enslow Publishers, 1998.

Willett, W. *Eat, Drink and be Healthy*. Simon & Shuster, 2001.

Wilson, J.D., and Braunwald, E. *Harrison's Principles of Internal Medicine*. McGraw-Hill, 2000.

Witt, C., and Brinkhaus, B. "Acupuncture in Patients with Osteoarthritis of the Knee." *Lancet*, 2005, July 19, 366(9480):136-43.

Woodward, S. *Classic Mediterranean Cookbook*. Dorling Kindersley, 1995.

A

Acapulco dressing *See* French dressings
Acetaminophen *See* medication, acetaminophen
Acid-forming foods, 99-100
        Arthritis and, 100
Acropolis salad *See* salads
Acupuncture, 4, 5, 11, 14, 16, 19, 40, 53, 67, 69, 70, 72, 94, 146-148, 150,
        166, 184, 186, 198, 265-266 *See also* Alternative medicine
        Conditions treated by, 154-157
        Finding a practitioner of, 157-158
        History of, 150-151
        Technique, 153
        Theory of, 151-153
Acute pain *See* pain, acute
Alcohol, 42, 46, 51, 70, 86, 90, 99, 109, 115, 118, 128, 131-134, 140, 157,
        165, 199, 234, 240, 251
Allergic reactions *See* Food allergies
Alternative medicine, 5, 11, 17, 21, 78, 80-81, 143-151, 158-159
        Resources for information on, 264-265
American blue cheese dressing *See* salad dressings and sauces
Anchovies
Anchovy sauce, 257
        Green sauce, 257
        Niçoise salad, 228
        Northern Greek sauce, 258
        Puttanesca pasta sauce, 216
        Tapenade, 214
Anchovy dressing *See* French dressings
Anchovy paste
        Anchovy dressing, 228
        New Orleans remoulade sauce for poultry, 227
Anchovy sauce *See* salad dressings and sauces
Anti-inflammatory drugs *See* medication, NSAIDs
Antioxidants, 15, 31-32, 35, 50, 52, 62, 65, 67, 72, 96-97, 104, 110-112,
        116-118, 121, 128, 130, 132-134, 136-137, 140-142, 174-175,
        180-184, 192, 210-213, 231, 233
        As supplements, 174-175
Apples
        Louisiana collard greens, 221
Arabic dressing *See* salad dressings and sauces
Argentinean sauce *See* salad dressings and sauces
Arthritis *See also* joints
        Alternative therapies for, 148-162
        Bursitis and, 73

Arthritis *(continued)*
    Cartilage and *See* cartilage, arthritis and
    Causes of, 22-23, 26-29, 31, 36, 38-39, 55-60, 63-64, 66, 75-78
    Classification of, 22-25
    Conventional treatments for, 19, 146
    Diet and, 98
    Diseases causing (Group B arthritis), 22-24
    Exercise and, 83-84, 93, 162
    Explanation of, 18
    Fatty acids and, 45-46
    Foods causing, 52, 128-129, 132, 139
    Free radicals and, 29, 35, 50-52, 65, 67
    Group B, 22-24
    History of, 25
    Inflammation and, 7, 15, 22-23, 25-26, 28, 31, 35-39
    Injury (Group A arthritis) and, 22-23
    Joint abuse and, 28
    Joint damage and, 36-40
    Nutrition and, 5-7, 13-16, 29-32, 34-35, 37
    Obesity and, 32, 51, 105, 125, 134, 144
    Repair of, 56, 71, 98, 111
    Risk factors for, 26-32
        Age and, 27
        Ethnicity and, 27
        Food allergies and, 30
        Genetics and, 26
        Minerals and, 30-31
        Nutrition and, 29-31
        Repetitive stress and, 32
        Spinal injury and, 32
        Weight and, 28-29
    Supplements for, 15, 163-175
    Tendons and, 21, 24, 33, 35, 37
Arthritis Foundation, 158, 187, 189, 197, 203, 263
Aspirin
    Inflammation and, 45
Aquatic therapy *See* physical therapy, modalities

B

B-complex *See* Vitamin B
Back pain *See* pain, neck and back
Balsamic vinegar *See* vinegar, balsamic

Basic salad dressing *See* salad dressings and sauces
Basil
>Bruschetta Romana, 214
>Green sauce, 257
>Herbed French dressing, 226
>Italian dressing, 226
>Mediterranean beans, 223
>Napoli sauce, 259
>New Orleans Creole salad, 225
>Pesto dressing, 256
>Pesto pasta sauce, 216
>Roma sauce, 260
Bay leaves
>Argentinean sauce, 257
>Dry herbal sauce, 258
Beans, black
>Cuban rice and beans, 218
Beans, kidney
>Mediterranean beans, 223
Beans, red
>Caribbean mango-bean salad, 225
Blood sugar, 45, 48, 175, 205, 239
>harmful effects of, 98-99
Blue cheese dressing *See* French dressings
Boron, 173
Boswellia serratia, 174
Bouillon, chicken
>Easy yellow rice, 220
Bread, 103, 118-199, 123-125, 128, 133, 139, 141, 214, 237, 239
Bromelain, 174, 184
Broth, beef
>Cuban rice and beans, 218
Broth, chicken
>Spanish chicken paella, 218
Broth, clear
>Kyoto sauce, 257
>Thai ginger sauce, 259
>Thai sauce, 259
Brown sugar *See* sugar, brown
Bruschetta Romana, 214
Bursitis, 7, 10, 21, 23, 24, 70, 73-76, 78, 147, 160, 182, 193, 195
>Supplements for, 182-183
Busy-Maria dressing *See* salad dressings and sauces

C

Caffeine, 46, 134
Cancer, 23, 123, 125, 135-136, 144, 154
    Eicosanoids and, 46-47, 50, 52, 63
    Mediterranean Diet and prevention of, 97, 102, 104
    Red wine and prevention of, 109-110
Candy, 99, 119, 125, 236
Capers
    Acropolis salad, 222
    New Orleans remoulade sauce for poultry, 227
    Roma sauce, 260
    Sicilian sauce for pasta, 215
    Tapenade (olive spread), 214
Carbohydrates, 30, 114, 117, 231
    Processed carbohydrates, 104, 123, 124-125, 128, 134, 209
        American diet and, 30, 237-241
        As a cause of free radicals, 30
Caribbean mango-bean salad *See* salads
Carrots
    Chicken fricassee, 227
Cartilage, 34-38
    Arthritis and, 21, 23-24, 26-32
    Supplements for, 169-172
Catsup *See* ketchup
Celery
Chicken fricassee, 227
Cereals, 119, 123-125, 129, 132, 134, 141, 237, 240
Cheese, blue
    American blue cheese dressing, 226
    Blue cheese dressing, 226
Cheese, feta
    Greek salad, 224
    Nadine's dressing, 256
    Southern Greek sauce, 258
Cheese, Parmesan
    Pesto dressing, 256
    Pesto pasta sauce, 216
    Roma sauce, 260
    Walnut couscous, 223
Chicken
    Chicken à la Mediterranean, 229
    Chicken fricassee, 227
    Cuban rice with chicken, 221
    Omega-3 fatty acid-enriched, 155

Chicken *(continued)*
    Spanish chicken paella, 218
Chicken à la Mediterranean, 229
Chicken fricassee, 227
Chili powder
    Busy-Maria dressing, 255
    Curry-Thai dressing, 254
    Fine seasonings pasta sauce, 215
    Jalisco dressing, 255
    Lorenzo sauce, 260
    Mexican dressing, 255
    Mexican salad, 222
    Panang sauce, 259
Red sauce, 257
    Spanish chicken paella, 218
    Thai ginger sauce, 259
Chili sauce
    Acapulco dressing, 228
Chinese dressing *See* salad dressings and sauces
Chinese fried rice *See* rice dishes
Chiropractic care, 3-5, 11, 14, 16, 19, 40, 53, 58, 62, 69-70, 72, 94, 146-148, 159, 166, 184, 186, 197, 265, 267 *See also* Alternative medicine
    Conditions treated by, 159-161
    Counseling and, 162
    Technique, 161-162
Chronic pain *See* pain, chronic
Cilantro
    Caribbean mango-bean salad, 225
    Green sauce, 257
    Jalisco dressing, 255
    Mexican dressing, 255
    Mexican salad, 222
    Moroccan couscous salad, 223
    Panang sauce, 259
    Salsa, Mexican pineapple, 222
    Spanish chicken paella, 218
    Thai sauce, 259
Chocolate, 115, 116
Cholesterol, 104, 108, 122, 129
    Eicosanoids and, 48-49
    Mediterranean diet and, 110-111
Chondroitin, 170, 179, 181-182, 184-185
    With glucosamine, 171-172
Coconut
    Thai rice, 219

Cod
      Fried fish and beer, 228
Cold therapy (cryotherapy) *See* physical therapy, modalities
Colitis, 49, 156, 160
      Inflammation and, 130, 136
      Jupiter Institute Omega Diet and, 231
Collard greens
      Louisiana collard greens, 221
Compression *See* physical therapy, modalities
Conventional medicine *See* medical treatment, conventional
Copper, 173
Corn, 30, 98-99, 104, 115, 117, 119, 123, 125, 128-129, 132-135, 138, 211, 237, 239
      Caribbean mango-bean salad, 225
      Mexican salad, 222
      Spanish chicken paella, 218
Corticosteroids *See* medication, corticosteroids
Cottage cheese
      In Jupiter Institute Omega Diet, 112, 139, 233, 243-246, 249, 251-252
Couscous, 223
      Moroccan couscous salad, 223
Couscous, walnut, 223
COX enzymes, 104-105
COX inhibitors *See* medication, NSAIDs
C-reactive protein, 105, 130
CRP *See* C-reactive protein
Cryotherapy *See* physical therapy, modalities
Cuban rice and beans *See* rice dishes
Cuban rice with chicken *See* rice dishes
Cucumber
      Greek salad, 224
      Moroccan couscous salad, 223
      New Orleans remoulade sauce for poultry, 227
      Niçoise salad, 228
Cumin powder
      Busy-Maria dressing, 255
      Caribbean mango-bean salad, 225
      Jalisco dressing, 255
      Mexican dressing, 255
      Mexican salad, 222
      Panang sauce, 259
      Red sauce, 257
      Salsa, Mexican pineapple, 222
      Spanish chicken paella, 218

Curry powder
	Curry sauce, 254
	Curry-Thai dressing, 254
	Fine seasonings pasta sauce, 215
	Jamaican rice, 220
	Panang sauce, 259
	Spanish chicken paella, 218
	Thai ginger sauce, 259
	Thai rice, 219
Curry sauce *See* salad dressings and sauces
Curry-Thai dressing *See* salad dressings and sauces

D

Dairy foods, 30, 42, 46, 98, 104, 112, 128, 132-133, 139, 179, 235
Degenerative disease, 9-10, 18, 20-21, 23-24, 26, 28, 31-32, 35, 38, 43, 59-60, 63, 75, 77, 108, 154, 161, 172, 174, 176, 186 *See also* arthritis.
Degenerative disk disease, 59
Diabetes, 23, 46, 97, 105, 122, 124-125, 128, 131, 134, 136, 144, 230-231, 240-241
	Free radicals and, 51-52
Diet
	Back or neck pain and, 122, 183
	Inflammation and, 45, 98-99, 107, 134-137
	Jupiter Institute Omega, 99-100
		Foods to avoid and, 97-99
		Fruit and, 101-102, 104, 106, 111, 116-118, 235
		Grains and, 101-103, 106, 114-115, 192, 234
		Menu choices
			Breakfast options, 244-246
			Dinner options, 248-251
			Snack options, 246-247
		Nuts and, 115, 234
		Olive oil and, 108-109, 114, 234
		Omega-3 fatty acids and, 104, 111-113, 118, 132, 134, 137, 235
		Recommended foods, 233-235
		Red wine and, 109-110, 115, 234
		Sauces, 215-216
		Vegetables and, 117, 235
		Weight loss and *See* weight loss
	Mediterranean, 100-112
		Antioxidants in, 110-111
		Benefits of, 102-104
		Cardiovascular health and, 104-107

Diet *(continued)*
 Mediterranean *(continued)*
  Foods important in, 108-112
 Mindset and, 231-232
 Processed foods and, 123-124, 126-127, 132-133
 Protein and, 102-105, 112-113, 132, 142, 231, 233, 242, 243, 248-251, 261
Digestive disorders, 20, 49, 55, 136, 156
Dijon mustard *see* mustard, dijon
Dill
 Dry herbal sauce, 258
 Italian dressing, 226
Dining out
 Jupiter Institute Omega Diet and, 251
Dry bean salad *See* salads
Dry herbal sauce *See* salad dressings and sauces
Dry Sicily sauce *See* salad dressings and sauces

E

Easy yellow rice *See* rice dishes
Easy-ones sauce *See* salad dressings and sauces
Education in physical therapy *See* physical therapy, modalities
Eggs, 30, 102, 138, 141, 214, 237, 243-245, 249, 251
 Louisiana collard greens, 221
 Omega-3 fatty acid-enriched, 137
Eicosanoids, 31-32, 35, 44-47, 51-52, 58, 61, 64-66, 70, 72, 85-89, 105, 107, 217
 American diet and, 66
 Jupiter Institute Diet and, 165-166, 170-174
 Mediterranean Diet and, 108, 127, 132, 134, 141
 Role of, 15, 38, 43-44, 48-50
Electrical stimulation *See* physical therapy, modalities
Enzymes
 As supplement, 174
Exercise, 13-14, 27-28, 40, 53, 60, 62, 67, 72, 74, 81, 83, 84, 93-94, 121, 130, 148, 162, 166, 186
 Benefits of, 187-188, 190-193
 Precautions and guidelines, 198-200
 Proper forms of, 193-195
 Therapeutic *See* physical therapy, modalities
 Types of, 196-197
  Aerobics, 196-197
  Flexibility, 196
  Sports, 197
  Strengthening, 196

F

Factory food *See* carbohydrates, processed; dining out
Fast food, 30, 32, 46, 51, 101, 132-134, 139, 212, 236, 240, 251
       See also dining out
Fat, saturated, 104, 123, 126-128, 132-133
Fatty acids *See* omega-3 fatty acids, omega-6 fatty acids, omega-9
Feta *See* cheese, feta
Fine herbs pasta sauce *See* sauces, pasta
Fine seasoning pasta sauce *See* sauces, pasta
Fish, 42, 96, 101-104, 106, 112-113, 118, 130, 134, 136, 173, 192
       Mercury contamination of, 120-121
           Omega-3 fatty acids and, 111-112, 128, 137-138, 175-177,
           179-183, 209, 211-212, 233-234, 241-242, 248-251, 261
Fish à la Mediterranean *See* Chicken à la Mediterranean
Fish oil
       As supplement, 111, 118, 130, 134, 175-176, 241, 261
Flaxseed, 115, 128, 130, 134, 137-138
       As supplement, 175
Flaxseed Oil, 118, 128, 130, 137, 175, 214
       As supplement, 176-177, 181, 183, 234, 241-242
Flour, 98-99, 125, 128, 132-134, 139, 214, 235, 239
Food allergies, 30, 32, 37
Free radicals, 6, 15, 65, 67, 97, 110-111, 131-132, 140-141, 210
       Antioxidants and, 50-52, 128, 174, 181, 192
       Causes of, 131-134, 140
       Effects of, 29, 35, 37, 135-136
       Supplements and, 167, 173, 177
French dressings
       Acapulco dressing, 228
       Anchovy dressing, 228
       Blue cheese dressing, 226
       French dressing, 226
       Herbed French dressing, 226
Fried fish and beer, 228
Fried foods, 51, 99, 109, 127, 134
Fruit, raw, 111, 116, 179, 211, 235 *See also* Jupiter Institute Omega
Diet, fruit
Fruit juice, 98, 128, 139, 240

G

Gamma-linoleic acid *See also* antioxidants
       As a supplement, 118, 131, 137, 175, 183
Garlic
       Argentinean sauce, 257
       Chinese fried rice, 220

Garlic *(continued)*
      Greek salad, 224
      Italian dressing, 226
      Jamaican rice, 220
      Mexican dressing, 255
      Napoli sauce, 259
      New Orleans Creole salad, 225
      Northern Greek sauce, 258
      Pesto pasta sauce, 216
      Puttanesca pasta sauce, 216
      Sicilian sauce for pasta, 215
      Sotogary dressing, 256
      Spanish chicken paella, 218
      Tapenade (olive spread), 214
Garlic powder
      Chicken à la Mediterranean, 229
      Cuban rice with chicken, 221
      Easy yellow rice, 220
      Panang sauce, 259
Ginger
      Chinese fried rice, 220
      Jamaican rice, 220
      Sotogary dressing, 256
      Sushi and sashimi, 229
      Taiwan ginger sauce, 255
      Thai ginger sauce, 259
      Thai rice, 219
      Thai sauce, 259
GLA *See* gamma-linoleic acid
Glucosamine, 15-16, 169-170, 179, 186, 192
      With chondroitin, 171-172, 181-182, 184-185
Grains
      as part of the Mediterranean Diet, 101-103, 106, 114-115, 192, 234
Greek salad *See* salads
Greek sauce *See* salad dressings and sauces
Green beans, 115
Green onion *See* onion, green
Green pepper *See* pepper, green
Green sauce *See* salad dressings and sauces
Group A arthritis *See* arthritis, Group A
Group B arthritis *See* arthritis, Group B

H

HDLs *See* cholesterol
Heart disease
 Alternative therapies and, 202
 Conventional Medicine and, 144
 Diet and, 99, 105-106 *See also* heart disease, Mediterranean diet and
 Eicosanoids and, 46-47
 Inflammation and, 135-136
 Medication and, 89
 Mediterranean diet and, 99, 101, 103
Heat therapy *See* physical therapy, modalities
Herbs, 101, 104, 111, 114, 116, 130, 134, 138, 140-141, 214, 235, 243, 248, 253, 260-261 *See also individual herbs*
 As supplement, 137, 174, 211, 266
 Recipes with
  Chicken à la Mediterranean, 229
  Jupiter Institute Omega Diet and, 256, 269
  Mediterranean herbal salad, 221
Herbed French dressing *See* French dressings
Horseradish
 Russian sauce, 260
Hot sauce
 Acapulco dressing, 228
 Cuban rice and beans, 218
 Curry-Thai dressing, 254
 Easy-ones sauce, 260
 Lorenzo sauce, 260
 New Orleans Creole salad, 225
 New Orleans sauce, 258
 Salsa, Mexican pineapple, 222
 Thai ginger sauce, 259
 Thai rice, 219
Hummus, 132
 Arabic dressing, 255

I

Inflammation 7, 15, 25, 51-53, 66, 190 *See also* arthritis
 Acute injury and, 22-23, 36-38, 70-76, 180-184
 Back pain and, 62-65
 Causes of, 22-23, 26, 28, 31
 Conventional Medicine and, 79, 82, 84-92
 C-reactive protein and, 130-131
 Diet and, 95-97
 Diseases and, 135-136

Inflammation *(continued)*
    Eicosanoids and, 48-50
    Exercise and, 191-192, 196-197, 199
    Foods causing, 98-99, 124-129, 131-134, 217, 238-240
    Jupiter Institute Omega Diet and, 100, 103, 105, 121-123, 134-135
    Mediterranean Diet and, 107-111
    Neck pain and, 57-62
    Omega fatty acids and, 140, 175
    Process of, 35, 38-39
    Supplements for, 43-46, 169-172
    Symptoms of, 41
    Therapies to reduce, 150
Injury *See* pain, acute
    Supplements for, 180-184
Insulin, 48, 175, 190 *See also* diabetes
    Omega fatty acids and, 122
    Processed foods and, 125, 238-240
Integrative medicine, 11, 17, 39, 60, 71, 148-149 *See also* medical treatment, alternative medicine, treatment modalities
Iodine, 174
Iontophoresis *See* physical therapy, modalities
Iron, 173
Italian dressing *See* salad dressings and sauces

J

Jalisco dressing *See* salad dressings and sauces
Jamaican rice *See* rice dishes
Joints 5, 20-21 *See also* arthritis
    Abuse of, 28
    Biomechanics of, 33-35
    Diet and, 30, 32, 98, 103, 111, 122, 131-136
    Diseases of, 59
    Exercise and, 93, 191, 196-206
    Inflammation of, 49
    Injuries to, 36-38, 70-71, 73-76, 111
    Repair of, 8, 13-15, 38-40, 92-93, 231
    Sprains *See* sprains, joint
    Supplements for, 169-171, 173
Jupiter Institute Omega Diet *See* Diet, Jupiter Institute Omega

K

Ketchup
>Easy-ones sauce, 260
>Ketchup sauce, 255
>Russian sauce, 260
>Swiss sauce, 260

Ketchup sauce *See* salad dressings and sauces
Krafty sauce *See* salad dressings and sauces
Kyoto sauce *See* salad dressings and sauces

L

LDLs *see* cholesterol
Lemon juice
>Acropolis salad, 222
>Basic salad dressing, 274-275
>Chicken à la Mediterranean, 229
>French dressing, 226
>Greek salad, 224
>Italian dressing, 226
>Mediterranean beans, 223
>Moroccan couscous salad, 223
>Nadine's dressing, 256
>Tapenade (olive spread), 214

Lettuce
>Caribbean mango-bean salad, 225
>Greek salad, 224
>Mexican salad, 222.

Lettuce, Bibb
>Niçoise salad, 228

Lettuce, romaine
>Niçoise salad, 228

Ligaments, 8, 14-15, 54, 57, 59, 63, 70-73, 75, 93, 102
>Arthritis and, 21, 32-33, 35-37
>Diet and, 102, 132, 135, 231
>Exercise and, 191-192, 195-196, 199, 207
>Supplements and, 182
>Sprains *See* sprains, ligament

Lime juice
>Acropolis salad, 222
>Caribbean mango-bean salad, 225
>Mexican salad, 222
>Salsa, Mexican pineapple, 222

Lorenzo sauce *See* salad dressings and sauces
Louisiana collard greens, 221

M

Mackerel
      Fried fish and beer, 228
Magnesium, 173
Manganese, 173
Mango
      Caribbean mango-bean salad, 225
Margarine, 99, 119, 123, 133, 135, 138-139
Marjoram
      Dry bean salad, 224
      Dry herbal sauce, 258
      Fine herbs pasta sauce, 215
      Herbed French dressing, 226
      Moroccan couscous salad, 223
Massage *See* physical therapy, modalities
Mayonnaise, fat-free
      American blue cheese dressing, 226
      Curry sauce, 254
      Easy-ones sauce, 260
      Fried fish and beer, 228
      New Orleans remoulade sauce for poultry, 227
      Swiss sauce, 260
      Tomatoes espanioles, 224
Medical treatment *See also* alternative medicine, treatment modalities
      Conventional treatment, 4-6, 8-9, 11-12, 16-17, 143-146, 148-150, 152, 201
      Limitations of, 19-21, 58, 68, 78-81
      Resources for information on, 263-265
Medication *See also* aspirin
      Acetaminophen, 85-86, 91, 94
      Corticosteroids, 85, 91, 94
      In pain treatment, 84-92
      Muscle relaxants, 2, 19, 41, 58, 85, 92-93
      NSAIDs, 16, 85-91, 145, 169-171, 182
            COX inhibitors, 87-89
      Painkillers, 2, 4, 9-10, 12, 18, 56, 78, 80, 91-92
      Topical pain relievers, 92
      Types of, 84-85
Mediterranean beans, 223
Mediterranean bean salad *See* salads
Mediterranean Diet *See* Diet, Mediterranean
Mediterranean dressing *See* salad dressings and sauces
Mediterranean herbal salad *See* salads
Mercury *See* fish, mercury contamination of

Methylsulfonylmethane *See* MSM
Mexican dressing *See* salad dressings and sauces
Mexican pineapple salsa *See* salsa, Mexican pineapple
Mexican salad *See* salads
Milk *See* dairy foods
Minerals, 15, 30-31, 45, 47, 108, 112, 132
  As supplements, 116, 137, 163
Mint leaves
  Moroccan couscous salad, 223
  Thai ginger sauce, 259
  Thai sauce, 259
Mirin wine *See* wine, Mirin
Moroccan couscous salad *See* salads
MSM (Methylsulfonylmethane), 172, 179, 183-184 *See also* supplements, cartilage-building
Muscles
  Arthritis and, 21-22, 32, 37, 75-76
  Inflamed, 13, 32
  Relaxants *See* medications, muscle relaxants
  Therapies for, 82-83
  Torn and pulled, 24, 57-58, 70-71, 73, 77
Mushrooms
  Chicken fricassee, 227
Mustard powder
  French dressing, 226
  Herbed French dressing, 226
  Kyoto sauce, 257
  New Orleans Creole salad, 225
  Swiss sauce, 260
Mustard, Dijon
  Mustard dressing, 254
  New Orleans remoulade sauce for poultry, 227
  Sotogary dressing, 256
  Tapenade (olive spread), 214
Mustard dressing *See* salad dressings and sauces

N

Nadine's dressing *See* salad dressings and sauces
Napoli sauce *See* salad dressings and sauces
Narcotics *See* medication, painkillers
Naturopathy *See also* Alternative medicine
  Resources for information on, 267
Neck pain *See* pain, neck and back

Neuralgia, 55
    Alternative treatment for, 123, 154, 161
Neuritic pain *See* neuralgia
Neuritis *See* neuropathy
Neuropathy 55, 60, 65
    Alternative treatment for, 107, 154, 161
    Supplements for, 175, 181
New Orleans Creole salad *See* salads
New Orleans remoulade sauce for poultry *See* sauces
New Orleans sauce *See* salad dressings and sauces
Niçoise salad *See* salads
Northern Greek sauce *See* salad dressings and sauces
NSAIDs *See* medication, NSAIDs
Nutrient therapy *See* supplements, nutrient therapy using
Nutrition, 5-7, 11, 13-17, 19, 29-32, 44, 58, 61, 64, 94, 95-97, 100, 146-148, 159, 162, 179, 186
    Anti-inflammatory, 192, 197, 208
    Effects of poor, 34-35, 37, 52, 131-132, 135, 139, 165-166
    Studies on, 188
Nutritional supplements *See* supplements
Nuts, 98, 102-104, 106, 118-119, 130, 134, 192
    Omega-3 fatty acids in, 115, 128, 137-139, 141, 175-176, 211, 241

O

Obesity *See also* Weight loss 4, 51, 105, 125, 134, 144, 232, 240-242
    Arthritis and, 32
    Exercise and, 191
Olive oil, 101-102, 108-110, 112-114, 116, 118, 128, 130-131, 134-135, 137-139, 141, 175, 179, 183, 209-213, 214, 217, 234, 241-242
    Acapulco dressing, 228
    Acropolis salad, 222
    American blue cheese dressing, 226
    Anchovy dressing, 228
    Basic salad dressing, 275
    Blue cheese dressing, 226
    Bruschetta Romana, 214
    Caribbean mango-bean salad, 225
    Chicken à la Mediterranean, 229
    Chicken fricassee, 227
    Chinese fried rice, 220
    Couscous, 223
    Cuban rice and beans, 218
    Cuban rice with chicken, 221
    Easy yellow rice, 220

Olive oil *(continued)*
  Fine herbs pasta sauce, 215
  Fine seasonings pasta sauce, 215
  French dressing, 226
  Fried fish and beer, 228
  Greek salad, 224
  Italian dressing, 226
  Jamaican rice, 220
  Louisiana collard greens, 221
  Mediterranean beans, 223
  Mediterranean bean salad, 224
  Mediterranean herbal salad, 221
  Mexican salad, 222
  Moroccan couscous salad, 223
  Nadine's dressing, 256
  New Orleans Creole salad, 225
  New Orleans remoulade sauce for poultry, 227
  Omega-3 fatty acids in, 156
  Pesto pasta sauce, 216
  Puttanesca pasta sauce, 216
  Salsa, Mexican pineapple, 222
  Sicilian sauce for pasta, 215
  Simple salad, 221
  Spanish chicken paella, 218
  Steak and hamburger, 227
  Sushi and sashimi, 229
  Tapenade (olive spread), 214
  Thai rice, 219
  Tomatoes espanioles, 224
  Yaya's dressing, 256
Olives, black
  Acropolis salad, 222
  Basic salad dressing, 275
  Bruschetta Romana, 214
  Greek salad, 224
  Mediterranean dressing, 255
  Mediterranean dressing (2), 256
  Mexican salad, 222
  Niçoise salad, 228
  Northern Greek sauce, 258
  Puttanesca pasta sauce, 216
  Sicilian sauce for pasta, 215
  Southern Greek sauce, 258
  Tapenade (olive spread), 214

Olives, green
        Acropolis salad, 222
        Arabic dressing, 255
        Basic salad dressing, 275
        Greek salad, 224
        Mediterranean dressing, 255
        Mediterranean dressing (2), 256
        Napoli sauce, 259
        Southern Greek sauce, 258
        Tapenade (olive spread), 214
Omega fatty acids *See also* eicosanoids, Jupiter Institute Omega Diet,
omega fatty acids and
        As supplements, 72, 167, 175-177, 180-183, 192
        Omega-3 fatty acids, 5, 29-31, 45-47, 49
                Anti-inflammation diet and, 15-16, 62, 67, 97, 104,
                106-107, 112-113, 115, 117-118, 120-121, 128, 130-138,
                165, 208-214, 217, 231, 233-235, 244-245, 247
                Antioxidants and, 51-53, 111, 121-122
                Ratio to omega-6 fatty acids in diet, 51-53, 140-142
        Omega-6 fatty acids, 6, 108
                Arthritis, Injuries, and, 175
                Cholesterol and, 129-131
                Fats and, 127-129
                Inflammation and, 13, 45-47, 49, 51-53, 135-136, 138-140
                Processed carbohydrates and, 104, 124-125, 238-240
                Pro-inflammatory diet and, 31, 67, 97, 114-115, 118, 121,
                123, 132-135, 166, 209-213, 231, 233
        Omega-9 fatty acids, 67, 104, 106, 137, 183-184, 210-213, 217,
        227, 231, 233
                Arthritis and, 175
Onion
        Caribbean mango-bean salad, 225
        Chicken fricassee, 227
        Chinese fried rice, 220
        Dry Sicily sauce, 260
        Jalisco dressing, 255
        Jamaican rice, 220
        Mediterranean beans, 223
        Mediterranean dressing, 255
        Mediterranean dressing (2), 256
        Napoli sauce, 259
        New Orleans Creole salad, 225
        Northern Greek sauce, 258
        Puttanesca pasta sauce, 216
        Roma sauce, 260

Onion *(continued)*
    Salsa, Mexican pineapple, 222
    Sicilian sauce for pasta, 215
    Sotogary dressing, 256
    Spanish chicken paella, 218
Onion, green
    Moroccan couscous salad, 223
    Bruschetta Romana, 214
    Soy sauce dressing, 254
    Spanish chicken paella, 218
Onion, red
    Greek salad, 224
Onion powder
    Busy-Maria dressing, 255
    Fine seasonings pasta sauce, 215
    Mexican dressing, 255
    Red sauce, 257
Oregano
    Argentinean sauce, 257
    Dry bean salad, 224
    Dry herbal sauce, 258
    Dry Sicily sauce, 260
    Fine herbs pasta sauce, 215
    Italian dressing, 226
    Nadine's dressing, 256
    Napoli sauce, 259
    Northern Greek sauce, 258
    Puttanesca pasta sauce, 216
    Southern Greek sauce, 258
    Spanish chicken paella, 218
Osteoarthritis *See* arthritis

P

Paella *See rice dishes*
Pain, 1-6
    Acute injury and, 68-78
        Ligaments *See* ligaments
        Muscles *See* muscles
        Rotator cuff *See* Rotator cuff
        Sprains *See* sprains
        Tendonitis *See* tendons
        Treatment, 77-78
    Arm pain, 65-66, 180-181
    Arthritis and, 18-25, 34-38

Pain *(continued)*
      Chronic, 55-56, 166
      Conventional treatment of, 79-94
           Medications, 80, 84-93
      Exercise and, 187-191, 193-199, 201-207
      Foods causing, 98-99, 128-129, 132
      Foods preventing, 99-103, 107-108, 111, 121, 123, 208-209
      Indirect causes of, 75-77
      Inflammation and, 41-43, 45-46
      Neck and back, 54-67, 183-184
           Causes of, 55
           Degenerative disease and, 18-21, 23-24, 59-60
           Lower back pain, 62-65
           Sciatica, 65-66
           Supplements for, 163-164, 166-167, 169, 171-173, 175, 177
           Trauma and, 57-59
           Treatment of, 77-78
      Psychology and, 55-56, 205
      Resources for information on, 262-263
      Treatment programs, 7-15, 39-40, 66-67
           Alternative therapy 143, 145-148, 150-160
Painkillers *See* medication, painkillers
Panang sauce *See* salad dressings and sauces
Paprika
      Arabic dressing, 255
      Red sauce, 257
Parisienne sauce *See* salad dressings and sauces
Parmesan cheese *See* cheese, Parmesan
Parsley
      Argentinean sauce, 257
      Greek salad, 224
      Green sauce, 257
      Mediterranean dressing, 255
      Mediterranean dressing (2), 256
      Moroccan couscous salad, 223
      Napoli sauce, 259
      New Orleans remoulade sauce for poultry, 227
      Northern Greek sauce, 258
      Roma sauce, 260
Pasta, 136
Pasta sauces *See* sauces, pasta
Peanuts, 116, 146
      Panang sauce, 259
Peanut butter, 116

Peas, green
        Spanish chicken paella, 218
Pecans, 116
Pepper, black
        Acropolis salad, 222
        Basic salad dressing, 274-275
        Dry herbal sauce, 258
        French dressing, 226
        Herbed French dressing, 226
        Mediterranean beans, 223
Pepper, black *(continued)*
        Moroccan couscous salad, 223
        New Orleans Creole salad, 225
        Puttanesca pasta sauce, 216
        Salsa, Mexican pineapple, 222
        Spanish chicken paella, 218
        Tapenade (olive spread), 214
Pepper, green bell
        Greek salad, 224
        Green sauce, 257
        Jalisco dressing, 255
        Napoli sauce, 259
        Northern Greek sauce, 258
        Roma sauce, 260
        Spanish chicken paella, 218
Pepper, hot
        New Orleans sauce, 258
Pepper, red bell
        Greek salad, 224
        Jalisco dressing, 255
        Northern Greek sauce, 258
        Puttanesca pasta sauce, 216
        Red sauce, 257
        Roma sauce, 260
        Spanish chicken paella, 218
Pepper, white
        Dry herbal sauce, 258
        Puttanesca pasta sauce, 216
Pesto dressing *See* salad dressings and sauces
Pesto pasta sauce *See* sauces, pasta
Physical therapy, 1, 11, 13, 16, 40, 53, 58-59, 62, 66-67, 70-72, 77-78, 94, 145, 148, 162, 166, 184, 186, 195, 197, 264
        Modalities, 81-84
Pickles
        New Orleans remoulade sauce for poultry, 227

Pine nuts
        Sicilian sauce for pasta, 215
        Turkish raisin rice, 219
Pineapple
        Salsa, Mexican pineapple, 222
Popo's dressing *See* salad dressings and sauces
Processed foods, 123-125, 127, 132-133, 231, 237-238 *See also*
    carbohydrates, processed
        Jupiter Institute Omega Diet and avoidance of, 97-99
Prostaglandins *See* eicosanoids
Protein, 131-132, 192, 231 *See also* Jupiter Institute Omega Diet,
protein and
        Dietary sources of, 102-104, 112-113, 142, 233, 237, 242-243,
        248-251, 261
        In cartilage, 34-38, 89, 170
        Inflammation and, 41, 43-45, 61, 65
Puttanesca pasta sauce *See* sauces, pasta

R

Raisins
        Turkish raisin rice, 219
Recipes, 214-229, 253-260
Red meat, 98, 101, 126, 128, 133
Red pepper *See* pepper, red
Red sauce *See* salad dressings and sauces
Red wine *See* wine, red Rice *See* rice dishes Rice dishes
        Chinese fried rice, 220
        Cuban rice and beans, 218
        Cuban rice with chicken, 221
        Easy yellow rice, 220
        Jamaican rice, 220
        Spanish chicken paella, 218
        Thai rice, 219
        Turkish raisin rice, 219
Roma sauce *See* salad dressings and sauces
Rosemary
        Dry bean salad, 224
        Dry herbal sauce, 258
        Fine herbs pasta sauce, 215
        Greek salad, 224
        Mediterranean beans, 223
        Mediterranean dressing, 255
        Mediterranean dressing (2), 256
        Moroccan couscous salad, 223

Rosemary *(continued)*
>Northern Greek sauce, 258
>Southern Greek sauce, 258
Rotator cuff, 70-72, 78
Rum
>New Orleans sauce, 258
Russian sauce *See* salad dressings and sauces

S

Saffron *In recipes, yellow food color can be substituted*
>Easy yellow rice, 220
Spanish chicken paella, 218
Sake
>Chinese dressing, 255
>Teriyaki dressing, 256
Salads, 241-246, 248
>Acropolis salad, 222
>Caribbean mango-bean salad, 225
>Dry bean salad, 224
>Greek salad, 224
>Mediterranean bean salad, 224
>Mediterranean herbal salad, 221
>Mexican salad, 222
>Moroccan couscous salad, 223
>New Orleans Creole salad, 225
>Niçoise salad, 228
>Simple salad, 221
>Steak and hamburger, 227
Salad dressings and sauces *Note: add Basic salad dressing to all recipes.*
>American blue cheese dressing, 226
>Anchovy sauce, 257
>Arabic dressing, 255
>Argentinean sauce, 257
>Basic salad dressing, 274-275
>Busy-Maria dressing, 255
>Chinese dressing, 255
>Curry sauce, 254
>Curry-Thai dressing, 254
>Dry herbal sauce, 258
>Dry Sicily sauce, 260
>Easy-ones sauce, 260
>French dressing *See* French dressings
>Green sauce, 257
>Italian dressing, 226
>Jalisco dressing, 255

Salad dressings and sauces *(continued)*
    Ketchup sauce, 255
    Krafty sauce, 260
    Kyoto sauce, 257
    Lorenzo sauce, 260
    Mediterranean dressing, 255
    Mediterranean dressing (2), 256
    Mexican dressing, 255
    Mustard dressing, 254
    Nadine's dressing, 256
    Napoli sauce, 259
    New Orleans sauce, 258
    Northern Greek sauce, 258
    Panang sauce, 259
    Parisienne sauce, 260
    Pesto dressing, 256
    Popo's dressing, 256
    Red sauce, 257
    Roma sauce, 260
    Russian sauce, 260
    Salsa, Mexican pineapple, 222
    Sotogary dressing, 256
    Southern Greek sauce, 258
    Soy sauce dressing, 254
    Swiss sauce, 260
    Taiwan ginger sauce, 255
    Teriyaki dressing, 256
    Thai ginger sauce, 259
    Thai sauce, 259
    Yaya's dressing, 256
    Easy-ones sauce, 260
    Caribbean mango-bean salad, 225
Salsa, Mexican pineapple, 222
Salt *Note: use sea salt in recipes, See also* sea salt
    Acropolis salad, 222
    Basic salad dressing, 274-275
    Caribbean mango-bean salad, 225
    Chicken à la Mediterranean, 229
    Chicken fricassee, 227
    Cuban rice and beans, 218
    Cuban rice with chicken, 221
    Easy yellow rice, 220
    Fine herbs pasta sauce, 215
    Fine seasonings pasta sauce, 215
    French dressing, 226

Salt *(continued)*
    Herbed French dressing, 226
    Louisiana collard greens, 221
    Mediterranean beans, 223
    Mediterranean bean salad, 224
    Mexican salad, 222
    Moroccan couscous salad, 223
    New Orleans Creole salad, 225
    Pesto pasta sauce, 216
    Puttanesca pasta sauce, 216
    Salsa, Mexican pineapple, 222
    Sicilian sauce for pasta, 215
    Simple salad, 221
    Spanish chicken paella, 218
    Thai rice, 219
    Tomatoes espanioles, 224
    Turkish raisin rice, 219
    Yaya's dressing, 256
SAM-e, 172 *See also* supplements, cartilage-building
Sashimi *See* sushi and sashimi
Saturated fat *See* fat, saturated
Sauces *See also* salad dressings and sauces
    New Orleans remoulade sauce for poultry, 227
    Pasta, 235-238
        Fine herbs pasta sauce, 215
        Fine seasoning pasta sauce, 215
        Pesto pasta sauce, 216
        Puttanesca pasta sauce, 216
        Sicilian pasta sauce, 215
Sciatica *See* pain, arm
Sea salt
    Benefits of, 245, 248
Selenium, 173
Sesame oil, 119, 128
Short wave and microwave diathermy *See* physical therapy, modalities
Sicilian sauce *See* sauces, pasta
Simple salad *See* salads
Southern Greek sauce *See* salad dressings and sauces
Sotogary dressing *See* salad dressings and sauces
Sour cream, fat-free
    Mexican salad, 222
Soy sauce, 136
    Chinese dressing, 255
    Chinese fried rice, 220
    Jamaican rice, 220

Soy Sauce *(continued)*
  Kyoto sauce, 257
  Mustard dressing, 254
  Sotogary dressing, 256
  Soy sauce dressing, 254
  Sushi and sashimi, 229
  Taiwan ginger sauce, 255
  Teriyaki dressing, 256
  Thai ginger sauce, 259
Soy sauce dressing *See* salad dressings and sauces
Spanish chicken paella *See* rice dishes
Sprains, 13
  Acute, 182
  Joint, 73
  Ligament and tendon, 57, 72, 74, 78
  Neck, 69
Spreads, 235
Steak
  Steak and hamburger, 227
Steak salad *See* salads
Steroids *See* medication, corticosteroids
Stress, 27, 29, 46, 51, 64, 128-129, 131, 134, 140, 145, 157, 231
  Exercise and, 190, 196, 198, 201-202, 205-206
  Joints and, 37, 75
  Red wine and, 110
  Therapies for relieving, 147, 159
Stroke
  Alternative therapies and, 143, 156
  Cholesterol and, 129
  Eicosanoids and, 46, 48-49
  Inflammation and, 105, 135-136
  Mediterranean Diet and, 97, 101, 123
Sugar, 30, 51, 118, 128, 132-134, 139, 179, 236-237
  Blood sugar *See* Blood Sugar
  Harmful effects of, 98-99
  Recipes containing
    Basic salad dressing, 274-275
    New Orleans Creole salad, 225
Sugar, brown
  New Orleans sauce, 258
Supplements, 11, 13, 15-16, 18, 40, 62, 67, 72, 80, 96, 100
  Antioxidants as, 110-111, 140
  Cartilage-building, 169-175
  Conditions requiring, 182-184
  For inflammation, 130-131, 134

Supplements *(continued)*
    Injuries and, 180
    Jupiter Institute Omega Diet and, 118, 121
    Nutrient therapy using, 147-148, 243
    Omega fatty acids as, 177-184
    Recommended dosage, 177-184
    Reliability issues and, 184-186
    Role in healing, 163-164, 166, 192-193
    Weight loss, 245, 251
    Vitamins as, 167-169 *See also* vitamins
Surgery, 2, 20, 71, 77-78, 163
    Alternatives to, 150, 159
    Conventional medicine and, 81, 93
    Diet and, 103, 107
Sushi and sashimi, 229
Swiss sauce *See* salad dressings and sauces
Synovial fluid, 33-34

T

Taco sauce
    Easy-ones sauce, 260
Tahini
    Arabic dressing, 255
Tai chi, 147, 201-204
Taiwan ginger sauce *See* salad dressings and sauces
Tamari sauce
    Sotogary dressing, 256
Tapenade (olive spread), 214
Tarragon
    Dry herbal sauce, 258
    Mediterranean dressing, 255
    Mediterranean dressing (2), 256
    New Orleans remoulade sauce for poultry, 227
    Southern Greek sauce, 258
Tartar sauce
    Fried fish and beer, 228
Tendons, 8, 57, 66, 71, 73-76
    Arthritis and, 21-22, 24
    Tendonitis, 182
        Definition of, 33
        Diet and, 102, 122, 135, 231
        Exercise and, 191-192, 196, 198-200, 203, 207
        Inflammation and, 15, 35, 87
        Role of 37, 54
        Supplements for, 182-183

TENS *See* physical therapy, modalities
Teriyaki dressing *See* salad dressings and sauces
Thai ginger sauce *See* salad dressings and sauces
Thai rice *See* rice dishes
Thai sauce *See* salad dressings and sauces
Therapeutic exercise *See* physical therapy, modalities
Thyme
        Tomato
        Argentinean sauce, 257
        Dry bean salad, 224
        Dry herbal sauce, 258
        Dry Sicily sauce, 260
        Fine herbs pasta sauce, 215
        Fine seasonings pasta sauce, 215
        Herbed French dressing, 226
        Mediterranean dressing, 255
        Mediterranean dressing (2), 256
        Southern Greek sauce, 258
        Spanish chicken paella, 218
Tomato
        Bruschetta Romana, 214
        Caribbean mango-bean salad, 225
        Greek salad, 224
        Jalisco dressing, 255
        Mediterranean beans, 223
        Mediterranean dressing, 255
        Mediterranean dressing (2), 256
        Mexican dressing, 255
        Mexican salad, 222
        Moroccan couscous salad, 223
        Napoli sauce, 259
        New Orleans Creole salad, 225
        Niçoise salad, 228
        Red sauce, 257
        Roma sauce, 260
        Tomatoes espanioles, 224
Tomato, crushed
        Puttanesca pasta sauce, 216
Tomato paste
        Sicilian sauce for pasta, 215
Tomato sauce
        New Orleans Creole salad, 225
Tomato, sun-dried
        Puttanesca pasta sauce, 216
Tomatoes espanioles, 224

Topical pain relievers *See* medication, topical pain relievers

Traction *See* physical therapy, modalities

Trans fatty acids, 104, 123-125, 127-128, 133, 139, 238 *See also* processed foods

Transcutaneous Electrical Nerve Stimulator *See* physical therapy, modalities

Treatment modalities, 11-17 *See also* Medical treatment
    Alternative Therapies, 146-147
    Physical Therapies, 82-84

Tuna
    Tomatoes espanioles, 224

Turkey à la Mediterranean *See* Chicken à la Mediterranean

Turkish raisin rice *See* rice dishes

Turmeric
    Turkish raisin rice, 219

U

Ultrasound *See* physical therapy, modalities

V

Vegetables, 30-31, 101-104, 106, 111, 130-131, 164, 192, 209 *See also* Jupiter Institute Omega Diet, vegetables
    Antioxidants and, 174-175
    Jupiter Institute Omega Diet and, 112, 117, 130, 134, 137-138, 140, 211
    Nightshade, 98-99
    Omega fatty acids and, 175-177, 211-212, 235, 241
    Recipes containing:
        Acropolis salad, 222
        Chinese fried rice, 220
        Jamaican rice, 220
        Mediterranean bean salad, 224
        Mediterranean herbal salad, 221
        Mexican salad, 222
        Simple salad, 221
        Steak and hamburger, 227
    Vitamins, Minerals and, 173, 179
    Weight loss and, 231, 234

Vegetable oil, 103, 119, 124-125, 128, 132-134, 138-139

Vibration *See* physical therapy, modalities

Vinegar, 99, 133, 248, 253, 261
    Basic salad dressing, 274-275

Vinegar, balsamic
        Basic salad dressing, 275
        Puttanesca pasta sauce, 216
        Yaya's dressing, 256
Vinegar, red wine
        New Orleans Creole salad, 225
Vitamins *See also vitamins by name*, 40, 67, 192, 231, 243
        As antioxidants, 137
        Brand selection, 184-186
        Deficiency in Americans, 30-32, 35
        Excessive use of, 167-169
        Effects of deficiency, 29-30, 34-35, 37-38, 163-165
        Foods, herbs and, 108, 112, 116-118, 137
        For arthritis & injuries, 167-172, 180, 184
        Recommended dosages, 177-180
        Role in healing, 7, 10, 15-16, 100, 130, 132, 163-166
        Usage in treatment, 80, 111
Vitamin A, 165, 167, 175, 179, 183
Vitamin B, 165, 167-168, 175, 179-180, 183, 186, 192
        B-complex, 165, 167-168, 175, 177, 180, 183, 186, 192
Vitamin C, 165, 167-168, 175, 177, 180, 183, 186, 192
Vitamin D, 168, 180
Vitamin E, 108, 167-168, 175, 177, 180, 183

W

Walnuts, 115, 118, 128, 130, 137-139, 141, 175-176, 211, 214, 241, 249-251, 254
        Acropolis salad, 222
        Basic salad dressing, 275
        Italian dressing, 226
        Pesto dressing, 256
        Pesto pasta sauce, 216
Walnut couscous, 223
Walnut couscous *See* couscous, walnut
Wasabi
        Sushi and sashimi, 229
Weight loss 69, 97
        Exercise and, 189
        Jupiter Institute Omega Diet and, 92
                Weight loss program in, 230-261
Wheat, 98, 119, 237, 239
        Allergies and, 30
WHCCAM, 148

White House Commission on Complementary and Alternative Medicine
See WHCCAM
Wine, Mirin
       Chinese dressing, 255
       Chinese fried rice, 220
       Jamaican rice, 220
       Kyoto sauce, 257
       Teriyaki dressing, 256
Wine, red, 42, 102, 106, 109-111, 115, 137, 140-141, 211-212, 217, 234, 240,
251 *See also* Jupiter Institute Omega Diet, red wine and
       Fried fish and beer, 228
       Parisienne sauce, 260
       Red sauce, 257
Wine, white, 109
       Acropolis salad, 222
       Anchovy sauce, 257
       Chicken fricassee, 227
       Cuban rice with chicken, 221
       Dry Sicily sauce, 260
       Green sauce, 257
       Italian dressing, 226
White wine *(continued)*
       Roma sauce, 260
       Spanish chicken paella, 218
       Tapenade (olive spread), 214
Worcestershire sauce
       Easy-ones sauce, 260
       New Orleans Creole salad, 225

Y

Yaya's dressing *See* salad dressings and sauces
Yeast, 30. 98
Yoga, 147, 201, 204-207
Yogurt
       Curry sauce, 254
       In Jupiter Institute Omega Diet, 102, 124-125, 139, 244-246,
       252-254

Z

Zinc, 31, 137, 173, 175, 180, 183-184

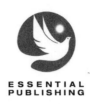

ESSENTIAL PUBLISHING

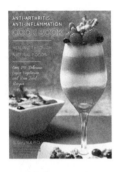

Anti-Arthritis, Anti-Inflammation Cookbook: Healing Through Natural Foods
by Gary Null, Ph.D.

This *New York Times* best-selling author brings you more than 270 anti-arthritis, anti-inflammation recipes to heal conditions and diseases of inflammation, which are largely perpetuated by the high-fat, high-sugar, chemically laden Standard American Diet (S.A.D.). Prevent and reverse diseases like arthritis, cancer, diabetes and heart disease by making the delicious offerings within this book the mainstay of a new eating program…your health and life depend on it!

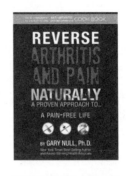

Reverse Arthritis & Pain Naturally: A proven approach to an anti-inflammatory, pain-free life
by Gary Null, Ph.D.

Arthritis is the most common cause of disability in the United States today, limiting the activities of a remarkable 50 million adults. Like cancer, diabetes and heart disease, arthritis is a disease of inflammation rooted in lifestyle choices. This book takes an in-depth look at the epidemic of arthritis and chronic pain sweeping our nation today, providing an explanation for its causes while offering a proven lifestyle protocol to reverse and prevent them naturally.

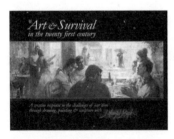

Art & Survival in the 21st Century: A creative response to the challenges of our time through drawing, painting & sculpture
by James Menzel Joseph

This art and social criticism book takes a profound look at the role of art in humanity's survival, and features over 200 exquisite and beautiful paintings and drawings of James Menzel Joseph, celebrated award-winning artist, author master art teacher, and activist.

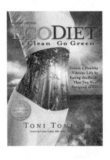

EcoDiet: Eat Clean, Go Green
by Toni Toney

Our connection to planet Earth is vaster than most of us realize. In fact, our body, like the earth, is an intricate ecosystem of interdependent organisms that depend upon one another to thrive. The balance of our ecosystem is delicate, and any disruption, such as an unsuitable food supply or a toxic overload, can damage or destroy it. In this important book, you will learn about the food choices that are creating an internal acid rain in your body – the cause of most disease – and how to restore balance and harmony.

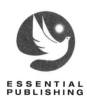

ESSENTIAL PUBLISHING

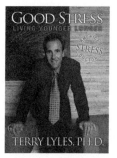

Good Stress: Living Younger Longer
by Terry Lyles, Ph.D.

Seeing stress as good is essential for achieving a youthful and vibrant life, says Dr. Terry Lyles, in this groundbreaking book inspired by years of rescue work at some the world's worst disasters: 9/11, Hurricane Katrina and the tsunami in Thailand. Dr. Lyles, known as America's Stress Doctor, implores us to see stress as a benevolent force. "If you want to live younger longer, start now by seeing stress for what it really is – a catalyst for positive growth and change.

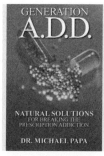

Generation A.D.D.: Natural Solutions for Breaking the Prescription Addiction
by Dr. Michael Papa

Free yourself and your children from the bonds of chemical dependency! In this timely and important book, Dr. Michael Papa urges us to explore and understand the symptoms and underlying causes of ADD/ADHD, and to choose natural solutions first, offering numerous approaches that have worked successfully with patients over the years.

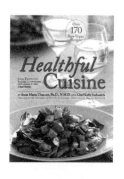

Healthful Cuisine – 2nd Edition
by Anna Maria Clement, Ph.D., N.M.D, L.N.C. and Kelly Serbonich

Learn about the superior health and nutritional benefits of raw and living foods from the world's #1 medical spa, Hippocrates Health Institute. This book contains: 150 raw and living food recipes, 40 pages of illustrated raw food preparation techniques, and more than 50 full-color photographs showing step-by-step instructions, plus tips from the experts. Making healthy raw foods has never been so easy.

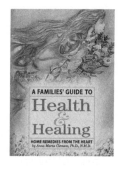

A Families Guide to Health & Healing: Home Remedies from the Heart
by Anna Maria Clement, Ph.D., N.M.D, L.N.C.

Bring healing back into the home! In this beautifully illustrated full color book, Dr. Anna Maria Clement, co-director of the world-famous Hippocrates Health Institute, show us how easy it can be to heal naturally with herbs, natural therapies, baths, flower remedies and aromatherapy. Contains more than 40 years of time-tested, clinical experience with natural healing modalities.